D0399266

Books by Ronald J. Glasser, M.D.

365 Days
Ward 402
The Body Is the Hero
The Greatest Battle

The Greatest Battle

The
Greatest
Battle

RONALD J. GLASSER,
M.D.

RANDOM HOUSE
New York

All rights reserved under International and Pan-American Copyright Conventions.
Published in the United States by Random House, Inc., New York, and simultaneously
in Canada by Random House of Canada Limited, Toronto.

Library of Congress Cataloging in Publication Data

Glasser, Ronald J
The greatest battle.

1. Cancer—Prevention. 2. Environmentally induced
diseases. I. Title.
RC268.G44   616.9'94'05   76-14200
ISBN 0-394-40018-6

Manufactured in the United States of America
9 8 7 6 5 4 3 2
First Edition

Preface

During the Christmas holidays last year, of the twenty-three children admitted to the largest pediatric ward of the University of Minnesota Hospitals in a single day, eighteen had cancer.

Cancer today strikes one out of every four Americans; two out of every three families. No one is spared, children no more than adults. This year alone, more than a million of us will begin treatments for malignancies. The death rate has been going up continuously. More people died of cancer in the first half of 1975 than in any other six-month period since the government began gathering nationwide mortality figures over forty-two years ago.

As alarming as these figures are, they are still misleading. The cancers we are seeing today did not begin yesterday or the day before, but twenty, thirty and even forty years ago. Scientists now agree that most adult malignancies have their beginning in childhood, adolescence and early adult life, some indeed even before birth.

Not everything, by any means, is known about the causes of cancer, but enough is known for physicians to say unequivocally that 75 to 85 percent of all cancers have nothing to do with viruses or even genetics, that they do not develop from trauma or because of infections, but result solely from exposure to environmental causes and industrial pollutants.

Where ignorance is to blame, who can be faulted? But often ignorance is not the case. The facts are known, they are available to every physician in the country, to every industry and government agency. They should be known to everyone.

For many of us, exposed for most of our lives, it may already be too late. But there is no reason why our children too should be doomed. There is still time to save them.

That is what this book is all about. The author is an instructor in pediatrics, a specialist in childhood kidney diseases, but mostly he is a pediatrician who realizes that the only real answer for disease is prevention, and prevention which begins in childhood, and that the lasting value of medicine has less to do with the development of newer treatments and more complicated machines than with its ability to prevent illness, to warn and to protect, and its willingness, for the sake of future patients, to admit and correct its own errors.

Today as yesterday the true reward for any physician, but especially for a pediatrician, is not the ability to prescribe or even to cure, but the simple elegance of not having to treat, of seeing all his patients grow up safe and healthy—of being able to live in the hope of never again having to stand helpless by the bedside as one after another of those he has sworn to protect close their eyes on those around them, and on all they might have been.

R.J.G.

Contents

The Greatest Battle

1

Our Modern Scourge

Cancer is today's plague, killing us and our children, our relatives and our friends the way cholera, diphtheria and smallpox once did. It is virtually epidemic. One out of every twelve women alive today will eventually have at least one breast removed. Tumors of the brain and bone marrow have replaced the terrors of meningitis and polio; the communal suffering and grief that were once the burden of such diseases as yellow fever, typhoid and tuberculosis now attend cancers of the larynx and bladder, malignancies of the liver and the lung.

This year alone some 80,000 Americans will be told by their physicians they have lung cancer. Some will be treated with high-dose radiation, others will undergo surgery, a few will be given drugs. But no matter what is done, almost none will survive twelve months. Next year 90,000 will be stricken, and the year after that, 100,000. In various degrees it is the same with most other cancers.

Why? It is not only the victims and their families who ask, but also those whose duty it is to pronounce the death sentences, and then try for a reprieve by removing a stomach, taking off a breast or opening a chest. Others, too, who have sworn to try to relieve human suffering ask why, the nurses who day and night must comfort the dying ask, the aides ask, and the orderlies.

So great is the problem today that every surgeon in the country may eventually have to admit, as one elderly surgeon recently did, that if the number of his own friends with cancer continues to increase at the present rate, he will be compelled, before his own death, to refer to other surgeons or to operate himself on just about everyone in the world he has ever cared about.

In 1976, at a national symposium of the American Cancer Society, a group of physicians tried to explain the why. Expecting to hear about the latest scientific breakthrough in the study of cancer viruses, or the development of a new anticancer drug, the audience was astonished instead to be told not to expect the remaining decades of this century to be a period of medical innovation for cancer or even of surgical triumphs but rather that the next two and a half decades will be the era of environmental disease, that the majority of all cancers are caused by environmental carcinogens, and that at a minimum 30 to 40 percent of today's malignancies could actually be eliminated by simply applying knowledge already known.

No mention was made of the need for better cancer research facilities or of bigger appropriations for larger detection and treatment centers. Instead, one after another of the world's greatest cancer specialists explained what a handful of physicians and scientists had been aware of for years: that the preponderance of malignancies are absolutely preventable, and that we can put an end to the scourge of cancer as surely and as completely as we eliminated smallpox and polio.

At the close of the meeting Dr. Irving J. Selikoff, director of Environmental Sciences at Mount Sinai Hospital in New

York, stated, "This session could not have been held ten years ago." The fact is that it could have been held at any time during the past twenty-five years, although few would have attended and even fewer would have listened.

To understand what brought about the symposium, why those in the forefront of cancer research and treatment now talked only of prevention and not of cures, of control rather than of vaccines, it is necessary to realize what has happened in medicine in the last century, its failures as well as the successes, and what has finally been learned about how malignancies develop and how they kill. It is an astonishing story filled with heartache and grief, blindness and corruption, self-service as well as self-sacrifice. It is a drama not of man against nature, but of man against himself.

II

A Tragic Medical Error

1.

The foundations for the symposium that Selikoff said could not have been held ten years ago was actually being laid as long ago as the late nineteen-forties. In those years, and continuing on well into the sixties, there took place in the United States what may yet develop into the greatest medically induced tragedy of all times. Through an error, first in medical judgment and then in medical prudence, hundreds of thousands of infants and young children were exposed to radiations that could someday cause their thyroids to become malignant.

In one city alone—Chicago—physicians estimate that at least 70,000 children were affected and are now, many years later, at the risk of developing cancer. So great is the medical concern, so widespread the problem that the Chicago medical establishment no longer was able to rely solely on itself but had to turn to the newspapers for help, not to alert people to the need for prevention or to generate support for public programs, but just to warn, to tell those at risk to come forward and perhaps be saved. In truth, by the time the newspapers were asked to help, it was too late for programs, too late for prevention. For those irradiated as infants or as children, the damage had already been done. What the physicians were doing by putting ads in the newspapers was trying to find the horse; the barn had been burned down decades before.

After World War II, irradiation of infants and of children became a way of life. The electronics industry, no longer involved in the war effort, had turned its prodigious energies to the domestic market. All the knowledge and production skills that had been gained in the development of the proximity fuse and sonar, all the technology that had gone into the delivery of thousands of reliable radar units were thrown into consumer products. Not only were electron microscopes manufactured, and electric eyes, but X-ray machines as well. They were turned out the way tanks and artillery had been, hundreds a month, and salesmen traveling across the country sold them. Within a few years after the end of the war there was an X-ray machine in practically every physician's office in the country.

X-rays became a routine part of office medicine. Sprains were X-rayed, hurt fingers, chests, backs, bones, abdomens, heads, necks. Enamored with their new technical ability to see inside the body, physicians began not only to X-ray almost every limb and every organ but to use their machines to follow the course of illnesses, taking X-ray after X-ray as viral pneumonias cleared, and greenstick fractures slowly healed. The ability to look inside a patient was unquestionably one of the major advances in the history of diagnostic medicine. The abuse of that ability was to become one of medicine's tragedies.

Hundreds of thousands of X-rays were taken every year, then every month. The mystique of the big machine, the conviction of the patient that he was being helped, a lack of understanding of what X-ray machines really did, neglect to read the available

literature on the dangers of radiation or refusal to accept what
no one wanted to believe—it is hard now to determine what
was most instrumental in the tremendous postwar growth of
the use of X-rays. By the late nineteen-forties, though, it took
only a very small step for physicians, already overusing their
machines, to turn up the voltage and begin to use them not
only for diagnosis but for treatments as well.

The average infant in America has between six to eight colds
a year. These colds or upper respiratory infections are annoying
but not serious affairs—a few days of stuffy nose, a little diarrhea, perhaps a slight fever, and the cold is gone. Mist tents,
vaporizers, decongestants, expectorants, aspirin or Tylenol,
used separately or together, afforded some relief, but eventually
the infant healed himself. That much at least was known back
in the late forties and early fifties.

But doctors, then as today, were reluctant to admit they
really didn't know what to do for these children, or perhaps
even more important, that nothing could be done. The use of
vaccines, the miracle of antibiotics, the development of even
newer surgical techniques, all have set the modern-day tone of
almost unlimited medical expectation. The public had learned,
or been taught, if not to expect everything from medicine, at
least to expect something, and physicians in large measure
responsible for that expectation felt obliged to satisfy that
general need. They felt even more obliged when it came to
their patients' children.

Patients don't like to be told they must get well on their
own, that nothing can be done, that it is simply a matter of
time and they'll be fine again. They like it even less where their
children are concerned. It is difficult to have an infant wheezing or coughing, difficult to stay up all night with a restless
child. Grandmothers get nervous when their grandchildren are
ill; neighbors and friends begin to wonder about parental com-
petence.

Parents want help for their sick children no matter what the cause, even if it is only a cold, and beginning in the late forties they got that help, or thought they did. What their children got was cancer.

2.

All children are born with a gland in the upper part of the chest called the thymus. In most infants it is large enough to be seen easily on almost any routine chest X-ray. The gland remains large for the first few months of life, then gradually decreases in size until the child is about a year old, by which time the gland has become so small that it can no longer be seen on chest films. Indeed, it shrinks so markedly during the course of the child's first year that it becomes almost microscopic, so small in fact that even during chest operations it cannot be found.

From the work of immunologists we know now that the thymus is one of the major glands involved with the development of the body's immune system. Its large size after birth is due to its enormous cellular activity during that time, when it alone of all the glands of the body gathers within it the millions of newly forming lymphocytes, turning those immature white cells into the killer T cells that we all need to defend ourselves from microbial attacks.

The body has always had a strict economy. Protected by our mother's immune system for the nine months of our forming, it is our hearts and lungs, brains and nerves, organs that we need even during fetal life, that develop first. Only near term as we approach the time when we must soon be able to defend ourselves out in the real world does our immune system begin to develop. So close is evolution geared to reality that the finishing touches are just being added when we are born. Yet our bodies, to be sure that we have the defenses we'll need to survive, keep the fetal organ that produces our immunologic system—the thymus—functioning even after birth. When finally everything is completely in order and functioning properly, when our immune system is completely developed, the thymus, its job done, is allowed to shrink away as the body begins to devote its resources no longer to protection but to growth and development.

The thymus, while it is putting the finishing touches on our immune system, is metabolically very active and like all such metabolically active glands is extremely sensitive to any type of radiation. Soon after X-ray machines came into general use it was discovered that the thymus could be shrunk artificially by exposing the gland to low-voltage radiations. Who it was that made the erroneous association between the number of colds infants have and their large thymus gland will never be known.

But looking back, we can now see how the reasoning connecting thymus size with the incidence of colds developed; why the idea was without the slightest proof so readily accepted by the medical profession. X-ray machines were universally available, thymuses could indeed be shrunk, and all infants were born with a large thymus gland in their chests. In accordance with the theory, treatment for colds were no more than a button push away, and physicians, wanting desperately to be able to treat their infant patients, unconditionally accepted the theory that the incidence of upper respiratory infections was related to thymus size. All over America, in institutions and hospitals, in large and small offices, in cities and towns, physicians began to put infants in front of their X-ray machines, turn up the voltage and direct the high-energy beams into the babies' chests.

Erroneous theories have always been a part of medicine. Ill-advised, fallacious, poorly thought out associations have continually occurred throughout its long history. The question is not why this occurs but why in this particular case it was so quickly and so widely accepted. The answer is not pleasant.

The association was accepted without any proof, without the slightest biological or medical reason to think there was a connection between thymus size and the incidence of colds, without any scientific ground to support the notion that shrinkage of the gland would in any way affect the severity or number of childhood colds, because the idea was simple and led directly to treatments with machines already available to every physician.

And the treatment became popular. Parents, tired of having their babies always fussy, and pleased that something could finally be done, happily brought their children by the thousands to the doctors' offices. And the physicians, catering to the parents' demands and proud themselves of being able to finally do something, cheerfully irradiated their young patients and collected their fees.

The fact is that the atrophy of the thymus in infants' chests and the decrease in childhood colds have absolutely nothing in common. They are two independent, totally unrelated events. The thymus gland shrinks when the body no longer needs it. The number of colds an infant has diminishes because his exposures to new viruses become fewer as he gets older. If the decrease in the number of colds an infant has is related to anything about the thymus, it is not to its shrinkage but to its large size—to the time when it is gathering together all the body's lymphocytes and turning them into killer T cells that will be used by the child to make his own fight, to decrease his own number of upper respiratory infections, to lead to the immunity that will indeed cut down on the incidence of colds.

Yet if irradiation was so effective, as was alleged, why stop with just treating colds? Why not use radiation for other conditions? And that is exactly what happened. In short order the

X-ray machines were used not only for shrinking thymus glands but for shrinking tonsils and adenoids in children, and then for treating acne in adolescents. Children now, not just infants, were put in front of X-ray machines and again there was potential disaster. By 1950, therapeutic low-voltage radiation had become almost a routine part of pediatric care.

In that year two physicians, B. J. Duffy and P. J. Fitzgerald, reported a disturbing observation in the prestigious *Journal of Clinical Endocrinology.* In an article titled "Cancer of the Thyroid in Children," they stated that of the twenty-eight children with thyroid cancer they had recently seen, nine had been irradiated for enlarged thymuses between their fourth and eighth months of life. (Two had already died by the time the report was published.)

Unaware of the danger of radiation, physicians had been casual about directing the X-rays. But even if they had tried to be precise about focusing the beams directly at the thymus in the infants' tiny chests, the tonsils in the throats of children, or the acne on the faces of adolescents, the rays would still have sprayed out. No matter what area of the head, neck or chest was irradiated, a few of the ionizing rays scattered enough to penetrate the thyroid gland developing in the child's neck.

Little attention was paid to Duffy and Fitzgerald's warning. The paper was not widely read, and even those who read it and were concerned ran into opposition. The article, it was argued, dealt with only a very small sample of patients. By the nineteen-fifties, thousands of infants had been irradiated. If there really was a problem from these low-voltage treatments, where were all the other children with cancer? Furthermore, how could Duffy and Fitzgerald be sure that the increased incidence they had observed in their irradiated patients was indeed caused by X-rays and not something else?

In 1952 R. C. Goldberg and I. L. Chalkoff, following up on

Duffy and Fitzgerald's work, publishing in *The American Medical Association Archives of Pathology,* proved that thyroid cancers could be induced in rats by the use of radioactive iodine and that thyroid cancers could be caused by irradiation. But physicians weren't about to stop treating patients on just "rat data." So the treatments continued, more children were irradiated and the incidence of thyroid cancers continued to increase.

3.

In 1955, five years after Duffy and Fitzgerald's warning and two years after Goldberg and Chalkoff's paper, Dr. Clark reported in the *Journal of the American Medical Association* that not only a third but all of the fifteen children he had recently seen with newly developed thyroid cancer had at some time in their early life received irradiation to the thymus, tonsils or other regions of the head or neck. In science as in everyday life, 100 percent of anything, even of a small sample, should be difficult to ignore. After Clark's publication, low-voltage X-ray treatments to the head and neck of children should have been stopped, at least until further studies; perhaps even a nationwide program evaluating all children already irradiated could have been instituted and the true risks of radiation determined before more children were exposed. But no such studies were made.

It must be kept in mind that the doctors who originally gave irradiation treatments believed in them, that they were not the ones who saw the cancers develop. The children left their offices healthy. It was other doctors, years later, who saw the real results of the treatments.

In part the problem was largely due to the distribution of

medical information. The majority of physicians do not read medical journals. It has been documented that if a doctor reads one medical journal, he will be the kind who scans them all; that a large number of physicians read none. This is even truer in the case of the specialty journals which reach an even smaller number of physicians. Most doctors in practice get their new information about medications and treatments from drug salesmen and company representatives. The dissemination of important medical facts without a wide-reaching publicity program, whether aimed at the lay public or physicians, is for the most part a painfully slow affair.

Despite the obvious importance of Clark's 1955 report, the practice of low-voltage X-ray treatments of children went on, in some places well into the late sixties. Infants and children continued to be put in front of X-ray machines, irradiated and sent home smiling, only to return to other physicians five, ten, twenty and thirty years later with cancers of the thyroid.

Finally in the late sixties, a full two decades after the first report of children developing thyroid cancers following low-voltage X-ray treatments, a whole series of medical and surgical articles relating the development of thyroid cancers to childhood irradiation began to appear in such numbers that the reports could no longer be ignored. But by then it was too late.

The first truly definitive paper dealing with the real dimensions of the problem appeared in 1970 in the *New England Journal of Medicine*. The article, evaluating a large number of patients, stated that fully 15 percent of all adults studied who had developed thyroid cancers between 1946 and 1968 had been given X-ray treatments to the chest in their early years. What made this study even more ominous was the malignant nature of tumors found in these patients. The article stated that the surgeons who had operated on some of these patients, a few immediately after the growths in the thyroids had been discovered, found that the cancer, even at these early stages of clinical discovery, had spread beyond the gland. Definitive pathological examination done on the removed thyroids found, time and again, even at operation, malignant thyroid cells already in the patients' blood vessels, implying that the operation may have been too late—cancer cells presumably even at the gland's removal already having spread to other parts of the body.

But that was only the beginning.

Three years later L. DeGroot and E. Paloyan, in their article published in the *Journal of the American Medical Association* titled "Thyroid Carcinoma and Radiation—A Chicago Epidemic," recorded their evaluation of fifty consecutive patients with thyroid cancer seen between 1968 and 1970, and reported that not 15 percent but as many as 40 percent of their adult patients had a prior history of irradiation to the head and neck.

Taken together, these articles presented an additional and perhaps even more frightening aspect to irradiation than simply the development of cancers. They indicated not only that the incidence of thyroid cancers following irradiation was increasing in the general population, but that the increase had doubled in just over ten years, the increase being made up by a continuing larger and larger percentage of people who had been irradiated as children.

In simplest terms; what this meant to the cancer specialist was that if you had been irradiated to the head or neck as an infant or child, your chance of developing thyroid cancer was very small in the first few years following treatment, but the chances mysteriously increased each year you lived even if you had never been irradiated again. The clinicians could not account for this increase, but their concern grew even greater when they began examining adult patients at risk because of such exposures in childhood, and found that physical examinations even of those adults designated "high risk" did not always in itself prove helpful. Cancers were found to develop suddenly in persons who just two or three years before had been examined and found at that time to be perfectly healthy.

4.

What was happening in these patients was something experimental cancer researchers had known for over fifty years: the development of overt cancers after exposure to any cancer-causing agent is directly related to the life span of the species exposed.

When experimental work on carcinogens—cancer-causing chemicals—began in the early years of this century, it soon became evident to the researchers that unlike infectious diseases, producing cancers experimentally was not an easy thing to do. The first attempts dealt with rubbing known cancer-causing compounds into the skins of animals, but notwithstanding lengthy applications, no tumors developed. Yet there was ample reason to assume they would.

In the eighteen-eighties Sir Percivall Pott, an English surgeon, related the skin cancers he found developing in chimney sweeps to these men's constant exposure to coal tars. From that time on, researchers in Europe and America tried to produce experimental cancers by rubbing those same tars on the skin of animals, yet no tumors developed. Even after weeks and sometimes months of continuous application, the skin remained normal.

But the Japanese, repeating the same experiments as their European and American colleagues and using the same kind of animals and the same carcinogenic compounds, continued the applications. Ignoring the world-wide ridicule of other cancer researchers, they continued to apply the compounds long after others had stopped. Daily they rubbed the coal tars into the same spot on the same part of their rabbits' ears, not for days, weeks or even months, but for years. Finally, with application times far exceeding any that had been tried before, cancers began to develop in the coal-tar-exposed areas.

With the publication of their report on the experimental production of cancer after long-term application of carcinogens, other researchers, following the Japanese methods, were themselves able to produce cancers. The long lag period between exposure to a carcinogenic (cancer-causing) compound and its production of cancer was found in experiment after experiment to be a universal physical fact. It did not matter what animals were used—rats, mice, rabbits, guinea pigs—the carcinogen or the method of carcinogenic exposure—spraying, ingestion, painting or injection. Cancers would not begin to appear until a time interval equal approximately to one-third the life span of the exposed animal had passed.

This common delay explained the reason for the long interval between the exposure of infants and children to low-voltage radiations and the development of their thyroid cancers. Cancer is above all else a cellular phenomenon. What applies to the cells of other living things applies to us. As a species we live approximately sixty years. The majority of people exposed to cancer-causing agents will begin to have their tissues turn malignant decades after exposure. This is what happened to the rabbits rubbed with coal tars and to the children exposed to irradiation of the head and neck.

Ionizing radiation is carcinogenic. We are now beginning to understand not only why this occurred but that indeed any kind of radiation can cause cancer. And with that understanding has come the growing uneasiness among scientists that there may very well be no lower limit of radiation exposure

necessary to produce malignancies, that any exposure to ionizing radiation may be dangerous. Of course, where the benefits
of radiation outweigh the risks, or where the risks are small in
relationship to the possible gain, exposures have to be tolerated.
As physicians and as a community we all, when ill or injured,
tolerate exposures to chest X-rays and skull films and to other
radiographic procedures—intravenous pyelograms, cholecysto-
grams and retrogrades—because the medical benefits are
deemed worth the exposure risks.

The real tragedy in the X-ray inductions of thyroid cancers
was that the treatments which exposed the developing thyroids
of a whole generation of infants and children to low-voltage
radiation were not only unnecessary but utterly worthless. No
scientific studies had even been done to prove there was an
association between enlarged thymuses and the colds of infancy, and no studies had been done to disprove it. Infants
were simply placed in front of X-ray machines and treated
because it was convenient.

Those children who had been irradiated for enlarged tonsils
had to be operated on anyway after the tonsils grew back, and
the acne of the adolescents returned. Yet X-ray treatments to
decrease the size of enlarged tonsils and adenoids, as well as to
shrink thymuses and control acne, continued to be used. Even
with a constant series of articles warning about the dangers of
childhood irradiation to the head and neck, the treatments
ceased totally only when the use of X-rays passed out of the
hands of the general practitioners into the hands of radiologists, specialists who had enough to do using their machines
appropriately without getting involved with the kind of un-
proven treatments other physicians had practiced.

Twenty-five years after they were begun, all such treatments
to the head and neck of infants and children finally stopped.
There will be no new cases of radiation-induced thyroid cancers in the next generation. But we still are faced with the

thyroid cancer of this generation and will be for the next thirty years.

The problem of those who had been irradiated as infants was brought into focus in 1975 with a publication entitled "Continuing Occurrence of Thyroid Carcinoma after Irradiation to the Neck in Infancy and Childhood," in which the authors, Refetoff and Harrison, unequivocally stated: "We are dealing with serious and potentially lethal tumors that justify an urgent surgical approach."

A whole generation was found to be at risk to develop cancers because of a carcinogenic exposure in infancy or childhood. It was no longer a matter of percentages or even the number of exposures; every adult who had been exposed or thought he had been was now at risk. At the very minimum the medical profession felt these people had to be continually observed, for the remainder of their lives, so that at the first sign of any abnormal growth or change in their thyroid they could be taken to the operating room to have the gland biopsied, and if need be, removed.

Concerned physicians across the country began the almost impossible task of trying to find the hundreds of thousands of adults who twenty and thirty years before had been exposed. Even where, as in Chicago, physicians enlisted the help of the mass media, only a few of those known to be at risk came forward to be examined. Many of those irradiated as children had already left the Chicago area and were at the time of the newspaper warning living unconcerned and unwarned in other states. Others who read the appeals in the newspapers could not remember if their mothers had taken them to a doctor or if they had been put in front of an X-ray machine and irradiated. Some knew they were at risk but because so much time had already passed and they were still healthy, they didn't care or weren't worried. They should have been.

Refetoff and Harrison concluded their article with this paragraph: "Comparison of these results with previously published studies confirms the risk of neck radiation in childhood and documents the highest prevalence (7 percent) of carcinoma yet reported. . . . The 100 patients included in our study received irradiation in 56 different institutions or independent offices. . . . If our sample of patients is representative, one would estimate 71,000 patients treated [as children] in the Chicago area only, indicating the proportion of the population at risk. It would not be surprising if this same situation exists in other cities. Radiation-associated thyroid carcinoma has not disappeared although at least 15 years have elapsed since irradiation for benign conditions of childhood and infancy was common practice."

It is obvious that the majority of people at risk have not come forward to be examined. They have read the articles and dismissed the warnings as applying to someone else, not realizing that it was the cells of their own thyroid gland that are involved, that someday they could be the ones to feel the lumps in their neck, the ones to be told they have cancer.

III

The Most Complicated Machine on Earth

We all begin life as one single cell formed by the union of the mother's egg with the father's sperm. The sperm, tiny fishlike cells deposited into the vaginal canal, propel themselves up through the cervical opening into the uterus. Sperm live for approximately three days, and all that time they continually move up over the uterine walls searching for the microscopic egg released by the female during ovulation. The egg itself lives only for approximately twenty-four hours.

It is essentially a race against time. The sperm have seventy-two hours to find the egg; the egg has twenty-four hours to be found. Using minute chemical and physical cues so delicate and fine that even today with our most sophisticated chemical analyzers and sensitive physical probes we are just beginning to discover not only that they exist but what the substances are, the sperm eventually track down the egg. Once they have found it, the sperm stick to the egg's surface, and one, using its tail to propel itself forward, forces itself through the egg's outer membrane into its interior, where the genetic material in the sperm's nucleus merges with the nucleus of the egg.

This single fertilized cell with its newly combined nucleus containing genetic material from both the father and the mother is all that is needed. This one single cell will, all by itself, given more than half a chance, with no other input, no other outside help, no additional information, turn itself in less than a year into the most complicated machine on earth—a new human.

Medical experts once thought, as many laymen still do to-day, that it is the organs of the body that are the basis of health and disease, that an injured heart causes heart disease and that infections of the brain lead to seizures and mental retardation, that digestion is done by the stomach and that hearing is accomplished by the ears. But early in the nineteenth century, with the use of the microscope, it was found that organs are themselves made up of different kinds of tissues and that the tissues in turn are made up of millions of even more fundamental units—cells. These cells, microscopic in size, made up of a nucleus containing the genetic material surrounded by a clear fluid called cytoplasm, were found to be the basis of biological life. You can divide the body into organs, the organs into tissues, the tissues into cells, but you can go no further without destroying life itself. We are, for all our intricacy, a structure built up from and maintained by these tiny basic building blocks.

Thousands of individual muscle cells pulling together enable us to run; the millions upon millions of red blood cells, each carrying a tiny amount of oxygen, deliver enough total oxygen to all parts of our body so that we can live. When the cells that make up the organs of our body function normally, we function normally. As long as the cells making up the retina of our eyes are healthy, we can see; as long as the cells lining the stomach continue to make gastric acid, we can digest our food. If, through injury, these cells can no longer function properly, can no longer do what they should, we become ill, the type of illness depending on the kind of cell injured as well as the type of injury itself. Destruction of the cells of our liver causes hepatitis; injury to a brain cell, confusion and coma; muscle-cell degeneration, weakness or paralysis. We know now that disease is not a bodily process, not an organ process or even a tissue process, but a cellular one.

To understand disease as well as health, physicians came to realize they had to understand cells and how they work. With the discovery that it was the trillions of cells in the body working together that allow us to do all the things we do, it was no longer adequate for physicians merely to feel an organ to make a diagnosis or smell someone's urine to tell what was wrong. To understand disease—why children are born deformed; why some people go blind and others bleed to death; why this brother gets diabetes and that one does not; why irradiation at four months of age leads to cancer thirty years later; even why there are malignancies at all, why even any illness—we have to understand our cells. But in order to do that, we must first understand how our cells come about, how they interact, what they are, what they are made of, how they develop, how they work, and finally, and perhaps most important, what controls them.

To understand disease we must first understand the process of life.

It was clear to the early embryologists, those scientists who study the development of life from the time of the union of the egg with the sperm to the birth of the fully developed child, that the first embryonic cell formed from the union of the mother's egg with the father's sperm must have within it, from the very moment of fertilization, every bit of information it would ever need to take it from that one single fertilized cell through its nine months of never-ending divisions up to the time of delivery when it finally had turned itself into a finished infant.

Unbelievable as it must have seemed to those early embryologists, they realized that the first cell had to have crammed inside its nucleus all the chemical and physical information necessary to tell it not only what to become but how to get there. Since every embryo unfolds from within, with nothing but nutrients ever added from the outside, those scientists had to accept the fact that the original single fertilized cell had to somehow "know" from the instant of conception how to transform itself into the billions and billions of ever more complicated cells that would eventually make up the tissues of the brain and the eyes, the muscles of the heart, the bones and the nerves of the new child.

At the beginning no one had any idea how it was done, what the information was, how it worked or even where in the cell it was stored. All they knew from the kind of changes that occurred was that the control was there, that it was in the nucleus, and that somehow the nuclear material told that single fertilized cell, and all the cells formed from it, exactly what to become, and somehow managed to take them there.

Using their microscopes to focus on the fertilized egg, the embryologists watched this unexplainable but magnificent transformation take place, watched bewildered and awed as the single fertilized cell sitting so quietly there in front of them suddenly and for no discernible reason began to quiver and then, under their very eyes, to divide. They watched as a whole microscopic universe with its own set of rules began to unfold as it had unfolded for well over a billion years.

In a kind of slow, almost painful throbbing the two cells became four, and the four, eight. The nucleus of each cell was duplicated, as were the cytoplasm and the cell walls. Where there were once 8 cells there were suddenly 16, where 16, 32. The 32 became 64, the 64, 128, the 128, 256, the 256, 512. By the end of one week the single fertilized cell had changed itself into a small ball of over 100 cells; by the end of two weeks, still no bigger than the size of a period on this page, the ball had grown to more than 600 cells.

Through their microscopes those early embryologists watched the tiny cluster of cells, each looking exactly like the one next to it, continue to divide, and then as the ball grew, with more cells being added, they saw the ball begin to bend and then gradually become elongated. If they could have looked closer, if they could have used the modern techniques of electron microscopy, or the newest fluorescent tissue stains, they would have seen that even at this primitive stage no two of those cells were actually alike, that even at forty-eight and seventy-two hours, indeed from the very moment of the first division, each newly formed cell was already beginning to differ from the one before. None was the same any more in size or shape, in cellular membranes and internal structures to the one beside it. The stunning fact was that although each two new cells were always formed directly from the same single preceding cell, just as that preceding cell was itself formed from the splitting of its own parent, no cell after the division was precisely like its brother or sister or even like its parent.

What presumably should have been an exact replica of the preceding cell was not. Each new cell had received exactly the same amount of nuclear material, the same amount of genetic information, of cytoplasm, exactly the same amount of cell wall as all the others, so that physically it should have been a precise replica with the same amount of internal information not only as its brother but of the original fertilized egg that had started it all. Yet each new cell, each coming from the same original cell and getting exactly the same amount of information as every other cell, was nevertheless internally and externally beginning to differ one from the other.

In ways that we do not yet understand, have not even begun to sense, the embryologists watched as each new cell, always containing the same genetic information in its nucleus as its predecessors, indeed as every cell around it, somehow began to use only certain parts of that information, and either not using or suppressing all the rest, slowly became its own unique self. Under the microscope, each cell, supposedly sitting next to its exact brother, became something totally different, this one slowly becoming a brain cell, that one being directed into forming a bone cell. Working at distances too small to be calculated, in amounts too tiny to be measured, chemical substances and physical triggers took over, and following the dictates of a world infinitely older than ourselves, allowed a new life to evolve.

The chemical and physical events going on within and between developing embryonic cells began in the first seas over two billion years ago; they began with the very beginnings of life and still continue today unchanged, so that sitting side by side, microscopically clumped together, no more than one thousandth of an inch apart, apparently the same and yet different, one fetal cell begins to develop fibrils on its way to becoming a muscle cell while its neighbor, destined to form a thyroid cell, starts assembling within it the endoplasmic reticulum that will someday manufacture the body's thyroid hormone. Every new division yields ever more cells, each new cell a bit more different, a bit more specialized, more individual than its predecessor, a bit closer to what that cell must eventually become so that the fetus when born can live on its own.

Precisely what the embryonic chemicals are that initiate individual cellular changes, exactly how they work, where they are made, how they diffuse out of one cell to affect those next to it, what physical forces are released from the cellular nuclei, what electric charges are dampened, which atoms are uncovered, how information from a cell's genetic material is translated into action or suppressed within the cell itself can only be guessed. Yet there is no doubt that these chemical events, mediated by minute but real chemical compounds, go on in and between cells in the same precisely regimented, well-defined, exactly reproducible way they have since life began. Indeed, it is because of these chemicals that life is maintained and prospers, that each new fertilization ends in a healthy individual.

Growing in all three directions, the ball of cells continues to divide; soon the numbers become astronomical. Where there were once 100,000 there are now suddenly 200,000; then 2 million; in the next instant, the 2 million become 4 million; within hours there are 8 million. The rapidly expanding mass of cells begins to turn and twist on itself, elongates and widens and then like a great pulsating wave folding in on itself, becomes a tube with an inside and an outside. Limb buds begin to form along the sides of the tube. Internally, right below the thin layer of expanding surface cells, a brain can be seen slowly to begin to form, a heart to be assembled.

In the midst of all these millions of dividing cells, one cell seemingly no different from the cell right next to it suddenly stops, and taking a chemical turn, begins to form itself into something new. Where a moment before there was no eye, a group of cells begins to form itself into one. In the midst of the developing brain, another cell, with no apparent outer manipulation, begins to change itself into one of the tiny nerve cells of our inner ear. A third cell near the growing limb bud begins to transform itself into the cell that will form the tissue which will eventually give rise to all our white cells and lymphocytes. A fourth, hidden deep down inside the mass of the embryo, begins to differentiate into the cell that will someday become our stomach; another into the cell that will eventually form our lungs.

The cells continue to divide, and by the fifth week each new division yields a cell not only more specialized and more internally sophisticated than its predecessor but also one with more chemical and physical abilities. Those cells beginning to form what will eventually become the muscles of the body not only elongate in shape, taking on a form different from all the other cells developing around them, but begin unlike any of their neighbors to acquire the ability to contract themselves. These fetal cells gradually acquire individual physical and chemical abilities that dazzle even today's most accomplished and sophisticated engineers.

Embryonic liver cells, dividing and differentiating right next to fetal bone cells, grow round and fat as they form within their cytoplasm tiny protein-making granules that will soon be manufacturing all of the body's proteins and fats, while bone cells shrink and begin to produce the solid substance that will be necessary to support us. In a world with borders no more than a quarter of an inch wide, a whole universe is being deliberately assembled. Cells that will form tendons stretch out and acquire the internal subcellular cables which will in nine months be able to hold bones together under stresses of thousands of pounds per square inch, while tiny nerve cells, unfolding less than a thousandth of an inch away, are turning themselves into electric generators, capable of discharging electrical impulses faster than a machine gun can fire.

For all the intricacy of what is going on, the seemingly independent development of these millions of dividing and differentiating cells, the apparent confusion of what appears under the microscope to be each cell type going off on its own, guided by its own special part of the total genetic information available within its nucleus, it is all still basically a physical process, initiated, maintained, organized and precisely controlled by chemical compounds, inducers, stabilizers, enzymes and potentiators which, while minute, are still as real and as physical as the earth we walk on and the air we breathe.

In the end it is these compounds and chemicals controlling cellular development, moving through and between the fetal cells, produced by them under the direction of their nucleic material at exactly the correct times and in precisely correct amounts, that drive it all. It is these compounds and chemicals that make fetal development possible. If anything happens to them or to their production, if the genetic information is injured, if the chemicals which transmit that information aren't manufactured on time, if they don't get out of the individual cells properly, if they don't fix to nearby cells in the right way, if the cells to be affected by these compounds aren't there, or the materials necessary for the next step of embryology to continue are not themselves ready and in the correct amounts, then there can be no orderly development. Then blood vessels will not develop where they should, muscles do not form in correct relationship to the bones, eyes wouldn't see. All normal development stops. We get disease then, and death, congenital malformations and lifelong disabilities. It is the same with cancer. What happens down at the cellular level of fetal cells to cause birth defects happens down at the cellular level of adult cells to cause cancer.

IV

What Is Cancer?

1.

Today we know that above all else cancer is a cellular disease. What causes it to develop happens down inside of individual cells, at the levels of molecules and membranes. Cancer is caused by injuries to minute subcellular structures; structures so small that they can barely be seen by our most powerful electron microscopes. We are just beginning to understand how these injuries occur and what the damaged structures are, and how, once injured, they can cause their cells to become malignant.

At a recent lecture given at the University of Minnesota, a world expert on the experimental production of cancer struggled to define for his scholarly audience exactly what cancer is. He had great difficulty and began first with what it isn't: "It is not simply the rapid growth of cells; the bone-marrow cells that make all our blood cells grow very rapidly. We completely replace all of our red blood cells every one hundred and twenty days, all our circulating white cells every six hours, and yet no one would say that this massive cellular turnover is cancerous."

He thought for a moment. "Indeed cancers, even among themselves, show a wide range of growth rates, from the very slow-growing tumors which do not produce symptoms for years after their known onset, to those that reach lethal size within a few weeks . . . Some of the most malignant and difficult-to-treat cancers are those that grow the slowest.

"Nor, for that matter," he went on, "are cancers restricted to just certain organs. They can and do arise from literally any kind of tissue cell. The opposite is also true—different kinds of malignancies can at times arise from the same exact tissue, each cancer, even though beginning from the same cell type, showing different biological properties. Some malignant cells can even appear totally identical to their still normal tissues of origin. Nor can you tell exactly how malignant a cancer might be from the form it takes. They can present themselves in any variety of cellular types ranging from a totally undifferentiated primitive-looking group of cells to a well-organized tumor practically identical to the still normal cells surrounding it.

"In most cases," he added quickly, "cancerous cells maintain some relationship to their tissue of origin, so that sometimes, even though malignant, they possess the functional abilities of the parent cells. For example, thyroid cancers may still produce thyroid hormone, even though the cells making the hormone are obviously malignant. With all this variation we now know that it is not the speed with which a cell divides, how fast it grows, what it does, nor what tissue it comes from that makes it cancerous, but it's independence. It is the lack of control over the way a cell divides and grows that makes it malignant."

Carefully choosing his words, the expert finally gave what with all his preceding qualifications was at least for him a precise if somewhat limited definition: "Cancer is an autonomous growth of tissue, no more, no less."

In other words, the definition finally presented to the audience was simply that tissues become cancerous when the cells that make them up no longer respond to the external, or their own internal, subcellular controls, controls that restrain them and keep them in balance with all the other cells of the body. Instead of dividing and forming more of themselves in a restrained and totally organized way, or simply staying where they are, and doing what they should do, making proteins, carrying hemoglobin, fighting infections or transporting fats, malignant cells take off on their own. Cells once docile and obedient begin to divide. Unrestrained, they begin to multiply, continually making more of themselves until their sheer numbers squeeze out the still normal cells around them; and then finally taking over the organ in which they first began. Eventually each new cell, an exact replica of the first malignantly transformed cell, breaks out into the bloodstream or lymphatics, spreading to the other organs of the body, lodging in them, taking them over as well. If the malignant cells undergo transformation in a necessary organ, like the brain or heart, the cancerous cells don't even leave the organ to kill the patient; they merely grow there until they interfere with some vital function like breathing or heartbeats, and the patient dies.

For other kinds of cancers the deaths are slower. A stomach filling up with malignant cells leads to nausea and vomiting and then starvation before the malignant stomach cells spreading to other organs causes death. Cancerous thyroid cells flooding into the kidneys crowd out normal kidney cells, causing the slow death of chronic renal failure and uremia. Nerves invaded by malignant breast cells produce excruciating pain long before the patient dies of disseminated tumor. Crippling pathological fractures caused by bones filling with metastatic cells may be the first sign of malignant lymphomas. Malignant cells invading lungs may cause asphyxia before they cause uncontrollable hemorrhage.

All the pain and all the sufferings of cancer come from the continual invasion of the body's still normal tissues by its own malignant cells. Cancerous cells, unrestrained by their own or any of the body's normal control mechanisms, go where they please, take over the body's energy and fuels when they want, and in the process squeeze out or starve the body's still healthy cells, causing not only the patient's death but eventually their own as well.

Today we know that cells are divisible, that each cell is made up of subcellular ultramicroscopic structures. We also know that these structures interact chemically and physically one with the other to keep a cell healthy, and that any injury to these structures, any interference with their communal microscopic interactions or control mechanisms, natural or man-made, is not only the cause of cancer, but basically the cause of all other illnesses as well.

2.

It is not that any of this is really new. It is only our understanding of what does and does not cause disease that has changed. Cancers have been noted since antiquity. Hippocrates and Galen, describing them under different names, wrote of malignancies two thousand years ago; Paracelsus gave classic descriptions of them well before the end of the sixteenth century. Livers turning malignant, lungs and stomachs eaten away have always been a horrifying part of medicine; they have been with us from the beginning. Yet until a few years ago no one knew what they were, where they came from, how they kill us.

Much of the confusion about what was and was not cancer, about spontaneous cures and remissions, almost all of the myths concerning treatments and prognosis, came about because for centuries cancers were confused with other diseases. Looked at superficially, even today leprosy can easily be mistaken for the slowly eroding squamous-cell carcinomas of the face and hands, echinococcal cysts for hepatomas of the liver, tuberculosis for lung cancer. Primary and secondary conditions only added to the confusion. Kidney stones found mixed in with kidney cancers were invoked as the cause for renal failure, while the blood and pus of meningitis often obscured small tumors of the brain. For centuries putrefaction was conjured up as the cause of liver enlargement rather than underlying cancers, while diseased arteries and veins were invoked for the tissue damage caused by infiltrating tumors or metastatic malignancies.

It was only when the microscope began to be used and precise microscopic evaluation of diseased organs and pathologic tissues became possible that the confusion about what was and what was not cancer finally began to be cleared up. There was no way under the microscope of making a mistake, no way any longer of confusing those wildly growing malignant cells with anything else. Physicians using their microscopes could definitively say this man died of cancer, that man of a bacterial infection. By the end of the nineteenth century pathologists were able, by looking at diseased tissues, to identify any number of malignancies by the type of cells that made them up—malignant melanomas, rhabdomyosarcomas, astrocytomas, adenocarcinomas, hepatomas. As their microscopic abilities improved, so did the number of diagnosed malignancies: osteogenic sarcomas, hypernephromas, oat-cell carcinomas, histocytosis. The list grew and grew.

But the names meant nothing. Patients died just as slowly and just as horribly with a correct diagnosis as those who had died misdiagnosed or with no diagnosis at all. The ability to recognize the various malignancies was only the beginning.

The real question was not the what or even the how of cancer, but the why. Yet the ability of anatomists finally to be able to say that in this case the primary cause of death was malignant melanoma, in that adenocarcinoma, gave physicians what they had been looking for: a place to begin. By the eighteen-nineties physicians were able for the first time in history to know exactly who had cancer and who did not and precisely what cell type was involved. No one then could have realized that the search for what caused these malignancies, the search that would give meaning to the names they were just beginning to catalogue, would take others down into the very heart of life itself; into chemistries almost too complicated to be dreamed of, into areas too small even to be seen.

3.

The experimental study of cancer began in 1901 when the Japanese researchers K. Yamagiwa and K. Ichikawa finally proved that skin malignancies would result from the continuous application of coal-tar preparations to what previously had been normal skin. For a quarter of a century the mechanisms that caused the exposed cells to become malignant remained unknown. Up until the nineteen-twenties all that was known about cancer was what the Japanese had already proved: that there were carcinogenic compounds which, when continually applied to tissues, would cause the cells of these tissues to become malignant. Today we know that what produces malignancies are the same events that cause fetal toxicities and congenital defects—cellular damage.

The original discovery which upset the theory that cancer production results from nothing more than a constant exposure of normal cells to a carcinogenic agent was made by Peyton

Rous in the early nineteen-twenties. Using the Japanese method for producing experimental cancers, he was painting rabbits' ears with coal-tar preparations, fully expecting to have to paint the same patch of skin for at least a year before any cancers became evident. Then, having to move his rabbits to another research area, he decided to renumber the animals by punching little holes in their ears so that they could still be identified even if there were two or three to a cage. To his surprise, cancers soon began to develop around the punch sites, months before any cancers were expected to be produced.

Rous's observation was to cancer research what Fleming's observation of the clear sites—the areas of nonbacterial growth surrounding the penicillin mold—was to infectious diseases, or Kukelel's dream of linked carbon atoms was to organic chemistry. The discovery that cancers would develop much earlier in normal skin exposed to a small amount of a known carcinogen if that skin was exposed to a second, in itself noncancer-causing insult, even one as seemingly innocuous as a tiny cut, led to development of the important concept of cancer inducers and cancer promoters. This concept of inducers and promoters is now central to the understanding of how cancers are produced, not only explaining what have been some of the most confusing aspects of cancer production, but pointing the way to an understanding of not only why cancers take so long to develop but why malignancies are themselves so deadly.

Following Rous's lead, researchers in short order found that they too could induce a similarly rapid production of cancers in coal-tar pre-treated skin by exposing these pre-treated tissues to almost any irritant, even by the simple application of turpentine to the coal-tar-exposed areas.

The implications of these discoveries were terrifying. The idea that small, virtually minuscule amounts of a known carcinogen—not the constant heavy exposure once thought necessary—could, if coupled or followed by some kind of irritant, produce cancers, had far-reaching implications. What it meant experimentally was that the total dose of carcinogen once considered necessary to cause the production of cancers was probably much lower than expected, and that the exposure time, if coupled with an appropriate irritating substance, could be reduced not only from years to months, but in some cases even to weeks. After the publication of Rous's and others' work on the production of malignancies, the real question facing cancer researchers was no longer whether chemicals could cause cancers, but exactly how long such exposures took, what exposure amounts were necessary, how carcinogens worked.

In 1940 Isaac Berenblum, one of our greatest cancer researchers of all time, beginning with Rous's observation, painstakingly set about to prove or disprove the crucial point of Rous's work—what was to become the crucial point of all cancer production—the precise importance of irritation. In short, he started out to discover what exactly the connection was between normal cells, carcinogens and irritants. Could irritants alone cause cancer and how, in the tiny world of cellular differentiation, could minute, not massive exposures to carcinogens cause normal cells to undergo malignant transformations?

He succeeded. Within a four-year period of virtually constant work he proved what industry today still refuses to acknowledge—namely, that small, even infinitesimal exposure of normal cells to cancer-causing chemicals can cause malignant transformations.

Using benzopyrene, a very potent carcinogen distilled from coal tars, Berenblum began his experiments by rubbing the chemical into the skin of hundreds of animals. Dividing the animals into groups, he constantly increased the concentration of the benzopyrene. Unlike the crude low-potency coal tar

Rous had used, only a few applications of the concentrated benzopyrene were necessary to produce malignancies.

Waiting to see which group of animals would develop skin cancers, Berenblum graphed out his results and found what he had expected, that the incidence of cancer production was related to the amount of benzopyrene applied to the skin cells. At very low concentrations of the chemical, no cancers developed in any of the exposed animals. It was only when the amount applied reached a certain high and seemingly critical level that the first cancers began to be produced. Once past that critical point, the number of animals developing skin cancers increased as the concentration of benzopyrene increased, until at very high concentrations of the carcinogen virtually every one of the animals developed skin malignancies.

But the truly important experiments were only now to begin. Berenblum realized he had really proved nothing with his increasing concentrations of benzopyrene that had not been known before. The real issue was not whether a carcinogen caused cells to become malignant—that was already known— but whether the cells of those animals exposed to a low concentration of a known carcinogen, in this case benzopyrene, those cells where the skin was exposed but still appeared perfectly healthy, had nevertheless been changed so that in fact the tissues were no longer normal. In short, did even minute exposure to carcinogens change the exposed cells internally so that despite looking and acting outwardly normal, they were really premalignant?

To find out, Berenblum went on to devise what has become one of the classic cancer experiments of modern times. It was an elegantly simple experiment, but it was to indicate the difference between life and death. Berenblum took the mice whose skin had been exposed to the low, apparently noncarcinogenic doses of benzopyrene and rubbed the skin with croton oil. It had been known for years that croton oil applied to normal skin would cause irritation and redness but never cancer. Yet when he rubbed the oil into the supposedly still healthy skin, it suddenly turned cancerous and the malignancies produced were indistinguishable from those produced in animals exposed only to high concentrations of benzopyrene. He repeated his experiments with other mice and found the same thing. He could at will reproducibly initiate cancers in supposedly still perfectly healthy, though carcinogenic-exposed skin by the addition of nothing more than an irritating solution.

It was plain to Berenblum and to others who read his report that the exposure of healthy cells to low dosages of a carcinogen, while not capable of causing overt malignancies itself, did nevertheless change the exposed cells so that subsequently what should have been no more than a simple innocuous irritation would cause them suddenly to undergo a cancerous transformation, the irritated tissues becoming overtly malignant.

Berenblum and the cancer researchers who followed his lead had to accept the fact that outwardly normal cells once exposed to a carcinogen were obviously no longer normal inside. The carcinogen absorbed by the cells, while not making them overtly malignant, had turned them instead into tiny time bombs ready to go off at what appeared to be the slightest provocation. These pre-exposed cells, rather than healing themselves after exposure to irritating substances as any normal healthy cell would, instead became frankly malignant.

By this time, two new scientific words—initiator and promoter—had been coined. The carcinogens which normal cells are exposed to are called the initiators, and the irritant causing the malignant transformation, the promoter.

More experiments followed. Instead of using relatively large doses of benzopyrene, Berenblum gave numerous small dosages. The results were always the same. While still appearing perfectly healthy, cells exposed to the small amounts of carcinogen would, when rubbed with an irritating promoter substance, become overtly malignant within days. The effect of the initiator was also found to be cumulative; exposures to the small, supposedly harmless amounts of a carcinogen did not have to be constant. They could be randomized with long periods between each additional small exposure, and yet the results never varied. When a critical small level of cellular contact was reached, the addition of an irritating substance resulted in cancer.

Berenblum made an even more ominous discovery, one that had to do with the time schemes involved. He soon found that no matter what he did, it always took exactly the same amount of time for a cancer to develop once the promoter was applied, no matter how long after the tissue had been exposed to the critical, though still outwardly noncancerous level of the carcinogen. He rubbed the skin with the low-critical, though apparently noncancer-producing concentration of the carcinogen and then waited days, weeks, months or even years before applying the irritant; yet no matter how long he waited, no matter how long the interval between exposure to the initiator and exposure to the promoter, the cancer always developed in the same amount of time following application of the promoter.

This meant that once a cell is exposed to a low but critical level of a carcinogen, it becomes premalignant and stays that way, never reverting back to normal, always ready on exposure to some irritant—no matter how long into the future, no matter how distant in time from its original contact with the premalignant levels of carcinogen—to turn overtly malignant. A cell exposed to a carcinogen was apparently not only a time bomb, but a time bomb that continued to tick and would continue to tick until either it died a natural death or, exposed to an appropriate irritant, turned cancerous.

4.

One thing became obvious at the very beginning of the studies of carcinogens and how they work. The changes which occur in exposed cells undergoing malignant transformations were irreversible; once transformed, the cells stay that way. Once cancerous, they never reverted back to normal. The development over the last few decades of the ever more radical cancer operations, the increasingly brutal mutilations practiced by surgeons and agreed to by patients as well as their families—the legs removed with the hip joints still attached, the radical mastectomies, the total gastrectomies—all are grim evidence of the reality of this fact. For cells that won't revert back to normal, that once turned fanatic stay fanatic, there can be no half measures and in most cases no measures at all. Remove not only the cancer but the whole lung of cancer patients, and 95 percent will still be dead within a year.

If just one malignant cell is left anywhere in the body, the cancer will recur. Malignant cells are relentless; leave just one cell and it is the same as not having removed any of the cancer at all. For some malignancies even the powerful anticancer drugs have proved ineffective.

It was plain to the first cancer researchers that cells which become malignant undergo some kind of profound and fundamental change. For these cells to defy treatments, never to revert back to normal, to continue to grow despite dosages of chemical poisons that could and did kill off the normal cells sitting right next to them, indicated that these cells were changed at their very core, in an absolute and profoundly fundamental way.

In the new specialty of subcellular research, filled with terms such as mixed function oxidase, enzymatic systems, proximate and ultimate carcinogens, free radicals and reactive substances, the facts of malignant and premalignant transformation become as evident as they are irreversible.

We now know that all carcinogenic substances, whatever they are, bind to intracellular particles, and the particles they bind strongest to and affect the most are the nucleoproteins contained in the nucleus of the cell—the DNA—the proteins that contain the genetic code. It is this DNA, holding within its own molecular arrangement the genes which tell the cell what it will be, what it will do and how it will do it, that is affected most by carcinogens.

In the chemical evolution that preceded life, it was these nucleoproteins that were the first molecules to reproduce themselves. Through the arrangement or coding of the bases, the sugars and phosphates that made up their own internal structure, these proteins eventually formed the materials of the first cells and then, taking their place within the center of these cells, the nucleus guided through the precise and regimented production of various minute, though distinct intracellular chemicals all future cellular evolution and cellular growth. The form of cells may have changed from the time of the first primeval seas, the nucleoproteins in their centers become more complicated, more sophisticated, intracellular structures and enzymes more intricate, but the control mechanisms of it all, the way the DNA and the cellular chemicals they produce direct and maintain both cellular form and function, have remained essentially the same through the ages. It is all still here today, all those controls, basically unchanged, two billion years later—locked away in the center of each cell.

It is only within the last few decades that we have begun to understand how the different arrangements of the molecules that form the DNA act as genes. Astonishing as it is, the only difference in genes, the only difference in the structure of a nucleoprotein that tells one cell to turn into part of the liver and another into part of the brain, that keeps this cell in the lymph node making antibodies and that one in the stomach making hydrochloric acid, that turns one fertilized egg into a fish and another into a child, is the sequences of the four simple carbon- and nitrogen-containing compounds which form the basic backbone of the DNA molecule: the bases adenine, guanine, cytosine and thymine. In a chemical code a billion years older than life itself, the arrangement of these bases directs like a master computer the way the cell's proteins are made and how they are put together, what the cell wall will look like, what the cell does, what it produces, and how it divides.

We know today, and it makes absolute biological sense, that it is the nucleoproteins, with their bases seemingly so safely for billions of years locked away inside the nucleus of cells, that carcinogens injure. It has been proved through a decade of precise, laboriously controlled research that no matter what the carcinogens, chemical or physical, no matter how diverse they may seem to be on the surface—benzopyrene or aniline dyes, asbestos or X-ray—they all share that one same basic property. They all affect the cell's genetic material by getting into the cell, and once inside, working their way into the nucleus, where they either bind to or simply destroy sections or parts of the cell's nucleic acids. We know that in large doses, carcinogens kill cells. They are all basically intracellular poisons. In smaller doses, because of their unique affinity for genetic material, they do not kill cells, they cause them to mutate, and it is this mutagenic nature of carcinogens that causes cancer.

If you take a hundred cells, grow them in tissue culture and

expose the whole culture dish to X-rays or immerse it in what
we know are carcinogenic compounds, you can, by increasing
the dose of radiation or the concentration of carcinogenic
material, kill every cell in the dish. But if you keep the doses
of radiation or carcinogen less than the amounts needed to kill
all the cells, a few cells in each of the culture mediums will
eventually turn malignant, assume unnatural shapes, and beginning to divide at unnatural rates, quickly overgrow the
whole culture dish. It is precisely what happens to the cells in
your own body when they are exposed to a carcinogen and turn
malignant.

There is nothing particularly mysterious about this. Carcinogens are toxic chemicals which are absorbed or diffuse into
cells. Once inside, they work their way or are carried to the
nucleus. There, in the submicroscopic world of cellular controls, one molecule of the carcinogen, or perhaps two or three
at the most, physically couples with the bases or perhaps even
the sugars of the nucleoproteins, and like a monkey wrench
jamming the control gears running a complicated factory, de-
stroys or interferes with two billion years of finely tuned evolution.

V

Old Plagues and Old Warnings

1.

As pediatricians we used to worry about children being born into a world of bacteria and viruses. Now we worry about them developing in a sea of chemicals.

The fears of drugs interfering with the cellular development of tissues, of medications getting into cells and poisoning their tiny internal structures, of minute amounts of environmental chemicals coupling with or destroying crucial intercellular proteins, of purely physical events damaging the intricate subcellular molecules necessary for normal cellular growth and development haunt not only pediatricians and embryologists but cancer researchers as well.

It should have come as no surprise to anyone, much less physicians, that the individual cells making up living tissues can be injured. In the nineteen-forties and fifties and for some physicians even well into the sixties, it may have been something of a surprise that cellular injuries could be induced by a supposedly harmless procedure such as X-rays, that the damage could be totally undetectable at the time of the injury and yet decades later could lead to those same injured cells becoming malignant. It may even have come as a surprise that cells exposed to minute amounts of chemical, even to cigarette smoke, could undergo malignant transformation, but certainly not that cellular injuries occurred and that those microscopic injuries could have horrible consequences.

Scientists have known for years that certain cells of the body could be poisoned, even killed, by literally infinitesimal amounts of materials not generally considered harmful and even at times known to be beneficial to the body. The knowledge of these cellular poisons is the result of a grim, though extensive scholarship, although one from which we seem to have learned very little.

Dicumarol, or bishydroxycoumarin, is an anticoagulant drug, a chemical extracted from the sweet-clover plant that interferes with the blood's ability to clot. It doesn't do this in the bloodstream, where we would expect it to work, but rather by getting into the liver cells which make the materials that clot the blood, interfering with those cells' ability to produce the circulating clotting factors. Taken orally, Dicumarol is quickly absorbed from the stomach into the bloodstream, where it circulates like any other absorbed substances to all parts of the body. The drug probably enters, at least to some degree, every one of the body's cells, but it is in the liver that it produces its effects. Liver cells differ not only in size and shape from all the other cells of the body but in the types of intracellular enzymes they contain. Liver cells and liver cells alone, because of their own unique embryonic development, are the only cells in the body which contain the protein enzymes that make the substances that allow our blood to clot.

The effectiveness of Dicumarol lies in its unique chemical structure, a molecular shape that somehow fits the structure of the enzymes in the liver cells that produce the circulating clotting factors. The drug's chemistry is such that once absorbed by the liver cells, Dicumarol interferes with only the cells' proteins that make the clotting factors and not with all the other enzymes in the liver cells, or for that matter any of the other enzymes in any of the other cells of the body. Given in correct amounts, the drug interferes with enough of the cells' clotting-producing enzymes to reduce the amount of circulating clotting factors, thinning the blood so that clots won't form, or even if they do, will not grow larger to block vessels or break free to cause heart attacks, strokes or sudden death. It is a very important drug for people with deep-vein thrombosis or pulmonary emboli, blood clots, and those with heart valves or dialysis shunts. But it is deadly to fetuses.

Dicumarol was first synthesized in 1942, and soon after, the drug and its derivatives were in extensive use in a wide variety of medical conditions. In 1945 the medical use of this drug was extended for the first time to treat predelivery thrombosis in pregnant women. There was no evaluation of the drug for use in pregnancy; it had worked in nonpregnant adults, so why not in pregnant women?

In 1947, two years after its beginning use in pregnant women, G. von Syndow reported the first neonatal death attributed to the drug. The baby was born dead and macerated, and showed a generalized bleeding tendency never seen before. The autopsy reported in Von Syndow's article was explicit. "Anatomical diagnosis: Massive hemorrhages of the thymus gland; focal hemorrhages of the lungs; bilateral hemothorax; hemopericardium; slight pulmonary aspiration of amniotic fluid; maceration with congestion and autolysis of all organs." Even reading the autopsy report today, it is obvious to anyone the least bit familiar with medicine that the child still being carried by its mother had bled to death by hemorrhaging into virtually every one of his internal organs.

Von Syndow ended his report: "Attention is drawn to the

dangers of fetal death from hemorrhage which may result from the administration of Dicumarol during the [predelivery] period."

There should not have been any need for the warning, not to mention the child's death. Twenty-three years before, in 1924, F. W. Schofield had published in the *Journal of the American Veterinary Medical Association* a report of a calf born from a cow fed sweet-clover hay; the calf developed severe hemorrhagic symptoms within a few hours after birth and died, while the mother remained healthy. Those who began to use Dicumarol in pregnant women should have known of Schofield's work; they should have checked the literature before they prescribed the drug during pregnancy. They should have evaluated the obvious association between the sweet-clover calf deaths and Dicumarol itself. They didn't.

Two years after Von Syndow's warning, J. J. Sack and J. S. Labote in the *American Journal of Obstetrics and Gynecology* reported another fetal death in utero of a child born to a mother who had received Dicumarol for thromboembolic disease. Post-mortem examination again showed a macerated fetus that had hemorrhaged to death. At approximately the same time Dr. A. J. Quick, a chemist concerned about the use of Dicumarol during pregnancy, performed the first experimental use of the drug in pregnant animals. Giving Dicumarol to a pregnant dog near term in dosages then being given to pregnant women, he reported that four of a litter of seven newborn puppies died because of hemorrhaging into their internal organs.

Yet in 1954, despite Quick's work, the use of Dicumarol was advocated for continued use in pregnant women. It was claimed that the drug could be used safely in pregnant women if the clotting factors of the mother were not lowered too greatly. It was the worst kind of wishful thinking, thinking that ignored scientific facts. In 1959 Epstein reported three more cases of intrauterine deaths associated with anticoagulant therapy, even where the recommendations of maintaining near normal maternal coagulation levels had been followed. In 1963 Mahairas and Weingold reviewed their own series of intrauterine deaths and finally stated definitively over a quarter of a century after Schofield's report that the drug should not be used for pregnant women in any amounts unless absolutely necessary to save the life of the mother.

The problem with Dicumarol was cellular injury.

When Dicumarol is used, a very delicate bodily balance has to be achieved between blood that will not clot easily and blood that will not clot at all. It is possible to give a patient too much of the drug, with the result that the amount which gets into the liver cells completely poisons all the clotting-factor-producing enzymes present so that no clotting factors will be made at all. When this happens the patient will be so "anticoagulated" that he will, like any hemophiliac, bleed from even smallest cut. People on inadequately adjusted levels of Dicumarol have bled to death from minor wounds, even from simple tooth extractions.

The disasters of this excess anticoagulation occurred early enough for physicians to know even in the nineteen-forties that every patient being treated with the drug had to have his blood continually monitored and the dosage of Dicumarol varied to maintain the correct and therapeutic amount of clotting factors. Yet the dosages that maintained ill persons without any excessive bleeding were the same as those that proved so disastrous when given to pregnant women.

Not only does Dicumarol affect a pregnant woman's liver cells, but crossing the placenta, it enters the developing liver cells of her fetus as well. By the fifth week of embryonic life,

substances in the mother's bloodstream are already entering
her baby's body. But the baby's body is more delicate than hers,
the enzymes in the newly developing cells more fragile, more
easily injured than her own. What is a medication for the
mother becomes a poison for the infant. Physicians can give
the right dose of Dicumarol to keep a mother's blood adequately anticoagulated, but for the child she is carrying it may
always be too much. With the enzymes in his liver cells totally
disrupted, no clotting factors at all enter his circulation. Even
as he is being carried, he slowly bleeds to death.

All through the forties and fifties the drug was given to
pregnant women the same way it was given to anyone else.
Despite the work of Quick and the isolated case reports of
human fetal deaths as well as the original animal studies, it was
thought that the placenta protected the developing fetus. In
spite of experimental studies and human case reports, the idea
of placental "protection" was still accepted. The theory then
current, with no basis at all except that physicians wanted to
believe it because it made treating their pregnant patients
easier, was that the placenta protects fetuses from all and any
dangerous substances in the maternal circulation. In some mi-
raculous way the placenta was supposed to keep out any medication given the mother, either destroying the drug or altering
it before it could enter her child's body. It took the continuing
deaths of children born with their lungs and brains destroyed
by hemorrhage, born having already bled to death, before
physicians began to realize they were wrong.

Irradiation of the thymus, giving Dicumarol to pregnant
women—X-ray treatments of acne and enlarged tonsils—each
of these was in a sense forgivable or at least excusable because
the majority of physicians who initiated these treatments did
not know they were dangerous. The real crime, the real culpability, what sensible men can only consider to be a total dis-

regard for common sense if not humanity itself, occurs when treatments are continued in spite of the reports and the articles alerting physicians to the dangers, or when new treatments are begun incorporating old errors. The terrible truth is that even after all the warnings concerning the anticoagulation of pregnant women, it took years for some physicians to stop prescribing Dicumarol during pregnancy, and well over a decade from the first reports on the dangers of irradiation to the head and neck to stop the use of radiation for treatment of benign conditions. The horror of all this, of infants and children wasted for no reason at all, of adults exposed or children having to worry the rest of their lives that their organs may turn cancerous, is that nothing essential has changed. Warnings about cellular poisons have continued to go unheeded.

2.

The idea of the placenta as a protective barrier was disproved once and for all by the deaths of the infants poisoned by Dicumarol. These deaths showed that there was a placental transfer of drugs, and while the deaths of these children eventually stopped physicians from prescribing anticoagulants to pregnant women, it did not stop them from prescribing other medications. It is hard to know why it didn't. To be harsh would be to say that modern physicians are prescribers, that the same pressures which made them turn up the voltage on their X-ray machines to shrink thymuses made them continue even after the disasters of Dicumarol to give drugs to women who were pregnant. To be more sympathetic would be to say that in a drug-oriented culture where treatment of some kind is demanded, where it is always easier to prescribe than talk, to treat than cure, doctors have simply taken the easier and expected road. But it can be the road of potential disaster and certain heartache.

It happened again with radioactive iodine. For people suffering from hyperthyroidism, an overproduction of thyroid hormone, the only permanent treatment available for years was surgical—removal of part of the gland itself. The gland was producing too much hormone and with no way to turn off this increased production, the only treatment available to physicians was removal of part of the gland so that what was left in the patient's body, even though overactive, would still be putting out normal amounts of the hormone. In mechanical terms the surgical treatment of hyperthyroidism was essentially the same as dealing with an overproductive factory by shutting down half or a third of it, and letting the remaining part, working at greater than normal capacity, produce what the whole plant normally functioning would have produced.

But the operation was risky. Hyperthyroid patients, because of their hypermetabolic state, did not tolerate surgery well, while just how much of the overactive gland to remove was always at best a wild guess. Some patients did indeed die at surgery, and some, having too little of their gland removed, had to be reoperated on, while others, having too much taken out, were forced to take thyroid supplements for the rest of their lives. Medical treatments were available, but they necessitated taking daily medications which had well-documented complications of their own.

The search for a truly definitive medical treatment for hyperactive-thyroid disease went on for years, a search that was unsuccessful until a radioactive isotope of iodine—I^{131}— finally became available at the atomic pile located near Oak Ridge. The reasoning that went into the use of a radioactive isotope for the treatment of hyperthyroidism was as elegant as it was ingenious. Physicians knew that normal dietary iodine is concentrated in a person's thyroid gland, where it is used by the thyroid's cells to make thyroid hormone. Since these events occur normally, the physicians treating hyperthyroid patients reasoned that a radioactive isotope of iodine would be treated by the body in exactly the same way as the naturally occurring substance. So close are isotopes to their natural elements that the body can be fooled into absorbing and using a radioactive element just as it would absorb and use the natural product.

Injected into the body, radioactive iodine begins to circulate along with the natural iodine. As the blood carrying the iodine passes through the thyroid gland, both the natural iodine and the radioactive isotope are taken up by the thyroid cells concentrated in them for use in the cells' manufacture of the body's thyroid hormone. Since the cells making up the thyroid gland are the only ones in the body that have the ability to extract iodine from the bloodstream, they are the only cells to be affected by the isotope's radioactivity. Small enough dosages can be calculated so that the injected amounts of radioactive isotope will injure only the cells that absorbed it, and no others, not even the cells lining the blood vessels that carried the isotope around the body.

What the thyroid researchers did in essence in developing radioactive iodine for the treatment of hyperthyroidism was to develop a tiny atomic bomb specifically designed to get into one and only one of the body's many cells and which, once inside, would emit enough deadly radiation to destroy the cell that had absorbed it. In reality, what physicians wanted to do with the isotope was to medically destroy rather than surgically remove enough of the thyroid gland to cure the disease. It worked. Physicians learned to inject just enough radioactive iodine to kill as many of the thyroid cells as necessary while sparing the rest.

With the development of radioactive iodine, internists as

well as surgeons began to treat patients with hyperthyroidism, and they did it painlessly, without the need for anesthesia and without the risks entailed in a surgical procedure. By carefully adjusting the dosage of the injected isotope, or by injecting small multiple dosages, the internists were able to get sufficient radioactive iodine into the overactive gland to kill just enough of its cells to bring the amount of circulating thyroid hormone down to normal levels. The decrease in the abnormally high levels of circulating hormone produced a gradual lowering of the symptoms of hyperthyroidism until finally, with normal levels achieved, the patient was healthy again.

But like natural iodine, radioactive iodine also crosses the placenta. At about the twelfth week of human embryonic development, the fetal thyroid gland begins to function. As far back as 1836, Jones described the microscopic structure of the human fetal thyroid. He placed its beginning of development at ten weeks following conception, but later, with better microscopic techniques and a clearer understanding of embryology, the time was put more precisely at between three and four weeks. At that time the immature cells in the fetus's neck which would eventually form themselves into a mature thyroid gland begin to gather together. Even at this early stage of development these cells are already beginning to differ from all the other fetal cells: their cytoplasm is a bit darker, their nuclei are a bit more elongated and slightly more off-center than those of the cells even right next to them. While other fetal cells are beginning to form the lungs and bone of the body, these cells, going their own way, acquiring the ability to absorb iodine from the bloodstream, develop into the thyroid gland.

In 1948, one year after radioactive iodine was made available for general diagnostic and therapeutic use, three physicians— E. M. Chapman, G. W. Corner and D. Robinson—began a cooperative study with the pathologists of Boston's Lying-in Hospital and the physicists at the Massachusetts Institute of Technology. This combined study was published in the *Journal of Clinical Endocrinology*. It was definitive because it dealt with humans, not animals.

"Pregnant women with organ diseases that endangered their health [and so for medical reasons were aborted] were given tracer dosages of radiation iodine from 12 to 48 hours before operation. At operation their intact fetus was obtained and carefully measured for approximation of age in weeks. The fetus was then fixed in formalin and sectioned longitudinally through the midline. Tissues from one half were prepared for microscopic evaluation while tissues from the other half were macerated in 5% potassium hydroxide for Geiger counter counts of radioactivity. Tissue was obtained from three levels: first from the upper pharynx down to the upper thorax, second from the upper thorax to the upper abdomen, and third from the upper abdomen to the lower abdomen."

What Chapman and his associates tried to accomplish was what concerned men of science have always tried to do: foresee the potential dangers in treatments that are being newly proposed, minimize the possible catastrophes and eliminate any unnecessary disasters. Specifically what they tried to do, anticipating the wide use of I^{131} and its eventual use in pregnant women, was find out at exactly what age of fetal development radioactive iodine would be damaging to fetal thyroids.

Tissues from nine fetuses were obtained. In those aged seven to twelve weeks the tissues containing thyroid did not exhibit radioactivity. In those fourteen to thirty-two weeks, the thyroid showed an amount of radioactivity that seemed to increase with each additional week of growth. Other tissues did not contain appreciable amounts of radioactivity.

In Chapman's own words: "Our studies indicate that the

human fetal thyroid does not collect administrated radioactive iodine in the first 12 weeks of life and that increasing amounts of radioactive iodine are collected after the fourteenth week. A practical application of this knowledge lies in the use of radioactive iodine in the treatment of toxic goiter hyperthyroidism. Women up to the fourth month of pregnancy may be given therapeutic doses of radioactive iodine without retention by the fetus." Put another way, by the twelfth week of fetal life the embryonic thyroid cells, in preparation for the thyroid hormone they will soon have to be making, have already matured enough to begin to be able to concentrate iodine.

What Chapman proved was that if at any time from the twelfth week of fetal life on a mother is given injections of radioactive iodine, the isotope will, like the natural iodine already in the bloodstream, cross the placenta and begin to be concentrated in the cells of her baby's newly developing thyroid gland as it is concentrating in her own thyroid cells.

In 1957, ten years after Chapman's report was published, two gynecologists, K. D. Russel and H. Rose, reported in the *Journal of Surgical Gynecology and Obstetrics* two cases of pregnant women, both of whom the year before had been given 25 to 225 milligrams of radioactive iodine. Both had either not been asked if they were pregnant, did not know they were, or had known but did not realize the treatments they were receiving would be dangerous to the babies they were carrying. Russel and Rose estimated that both women received the radioactive iodine somewhere after the thirteenth week of gestation.

In their article, the two physicians stated that both pregnancies proceeded uneventfully. The child born to the first woman, though, soon became severely hypothyroid. The second woman's child was delivered spontaneously at term and for a time seemed perfectly normal. Nothing remarkable appeared in the first days of the child's life except, as one of the nurses noted, "slow eating." At two months of age the second child developed a respiratory infection and mysteriously died.

The autopsy of this child showed no evidence of thyroid tissue. "Examination of the brain revealed some loss of nerve cells, with an indication that other [neurons] seem to be 'fading out.'" This loss of neurons, not death, was to be the real issue in infants' having their thyroids destroyed by their mothers' receiving radioactive iodine. As Russel and Rose stated: "The importance of the problem becomes especially urgent when one considers some aspects of congenital hypothyroidism (the destruction of the thyroid before birth). The physical effects of hypothyroidism are well known: large tongue, furrowed brow, thick skin, puffy eyes, constipation, poor feeding; less well known is the fact that there frequently may be a relative poor outcome in such patients with regard to mental development, even though [after birth] they might receive what is considered to be adequate [thyroid] replacement therapy."

Study after study had shown even before the use of radioactive iodine that retardation can result from hypothyroidism in infancy. R. E. Cook and E. B. Mann in an extensive study published before Russel and Rose's paper pointed out that although the general stigma of hypothyroidism could be well controlled with medication, the prognosis for normal mental development in hypothyroid children was poor. They found that none of the infants suffering from congenital hypothyroidism could be considered of equal mentality to that expected by the study of the rest of their families, even though the afflicted individuals in many cases received treatment considered adequate in regard to both early institution of thyroid hormone and total dosage. Many had intelligence quotients of less than 80.

We need our thyroid gland during fetal development for our brains to grow normally. If the gland is destroyed at any time during fetal development, the developing brain cells deprived of the thyroid hormone will never develop or function properly. It was not happenstance that the autopsy on the child who died of hypothyroidism in the Russel-Rose report showed no neurons in the brain. So definitive was their study concerning the irreparable damage to fetal cells following exposures to radioactive iodine that Russel and Rose ended their paper with the statement: "It will be noted that therapeutic termination of pregnancy may be considered in which large dosages of radioactive iodine have been utilized in pregnancies." What the authors were saying, in fact, was that it was better for the child whose mother had received the isotope to be aborted rather than to be born and live retarded.

We know enough today not to treat pregnant women with isotopes of iodine or to give them Dicumarol. Actually, we knew enough about radioactive iodine following the publication of Chapman's report in 1957, but because of confusion about risks, because doctors didn't ask the right questions or didn't believe Chapman's data, because patients weren't aware of the risks to themselves and their children, the treatment was given.

Always fewer in number, more fragile, more delicate than matured well-differentiated cells of an adult, the newly forming cells of a fetus are destroyed by the levels of toxic agents that are not harmful to adults and may even be beneficial.

The real problem with exposing fetuses to chemicals is not that fetal cells are more sensitive to both radioactivity and drugs than adult tissues but that in embryology there are no second chances. As physicians we have finally begun to understand that the stages of fetal development have been so intricately worked out, the evolutionary unfolding of one part of the embryo so closely meshed with the next, the times of cellular interactions so precise, amounts of tissue so deliberately balanced that any mistake, any error at any place or at any time during embryological development is a mistake forever. Every embryonic cell is programmed from its beginning to form certain parts of the body. Once those cells are lost or destroyed, they are gone forever. The economy of fetal growth is so rigid that there will be no others to take their place.

It is an understanding of that economy and the controls which maintain and run it that have led to the understanding of not only fetal poisonings and congenital defects but why mature cells turn malignant.

3.

Any physical injury to a fetal cell, any disruption of its subcellular structures, any interference or poisoning of any of its internal molecules, its carrier enzymes, its DNA or RNA, will result in congenital malformations. We are aware of this now, not because of what happened with Dicumarol or radioactive iodine—for all their grotesqueness these disasters, because of the small numbers involved, have remained relatively obscure tragedies—but because of the thousands of bright-eyed infants born without arms and legs. You might be able to ignore a few infants born hemorrhaging to death, or five or six left retarded from hypothyroidism. It was impossible to ignore schoolrooms filled with children trying to pick up pencils with their toes or little girls learning how to write with their teeth.

It was not physicians or their treatments who alerted the world to the cellular basis of disease, it was the drug companies.

Thalidomide was first synthesized in Germany in 1953. Its chemical structure was similar to but not exactly the same as what were at the time some of the world's best-known sedatives and mood-changers. The hope of the German pharmaceutical house in developing thalidomide was to make a new drug whose basic molecular configuration had already proved commercially successful, and then promote the new product into a highly profitable central-nervous-system depressant or tranquilizer.

Initially thalidomide did not prove particularly promising for either. It was not a very good depressant, nor for that matter a very good tranquilizer. Therapeutically it had little effect even when fed to adult animals. In various human screening tests, however, it did prove, when used as an anticonvulsant, to have some minor sedative effects, but nothing more. But this slight sedation effect was enough for the German pharmaceutical house to decide to push the new drug as a sleeping pill.

The first human toxicity studies on thalidomide were begun in the mid-fifties. To the growing excitement of the German manufacturer, it proved even in extremely large dosages to be almost entirely nontoxic. Unlike all other known sedatives, even in overdoses it did not suppress respiration, nor did it depress heart rates, two of the most feared and dangerous complications of sedatives. With the data about overdosing in hand and practically no further testing, the drug was released as a sleeping pill, and for a short time, at least in Germany, because of its supposedly wide margin of safety, was even allowed by the German government to be sold over the counter as a nonprescription medication. In advertising campaigns and sales promotions the drug company boasted of the fact that even those who had used the drug to try to commit suicide had not been able to kill themselves. Indeed, one intended victim was reported to have taken as much as 144 times the recommended dose and still survived.

With the growing success of the drug in Europe, two American companies began investigating it for use in the United States. The first company lost interest after conducting the same animal experiments that had been conducted in Germany. The firm concluded from its studies that the drug was worthless, and stopped any further testing of it. The other company, thinking the drug might be useful as a potential tranquilizer, subjected it to a brief human trial and concluded that it offered nothing over the other tranquilizers the company already had on the market, and so that firm, too, dropped it.

Two years later, in 1959, the American-based William S. Merrell pharmaceutical firm took thalidomide off the shelf and began another series of tests. In the years between the first testing of the drug by the original American firms and its resurrection by Merrell, it had begun to be used extensively in European countries other than Germany. With its growing European success the drug might, Merrell felt, still be potentially useful in North America.

Under the Merrell label, thalidomide was released for prescription use in Canada. But because of U.S. government concerns regarding some European evidence of the occurrence of bizarre and unexplainable neurological problems in long-term users, the drug was released in America only on a restricted basis, for use as part of a small clinical human trial. That was the status of the drug in this country when the pharmaceutical world fell apart under the combined weight of almost ten thousand children born without limbs.

In an ironic way, what happened to those thousands of children was so grim, so grotesque that it saved the pharmaceutical industry. Had the tragedy been any greater, become more widespread, world-wide anger would have been so overwhelming, the outcry of shocked and angry parents and friends for governmental control of an industry that could and did ruin children so shrill and unrelenting that the drug industry as it was then might have been abolished by such stringent regulations and restrictions that the companies would have become nothing more than distributors for government-developed medications.

What saved the industry was that the disaster it brought was big enough to hurt and lead to some changes but small enough to let its companies continue on, still basically intact, much the same as it had always been.

Only about ten thousand children were ruined, though you would have to talk to the parents of those children to see what the word "only" means, or even the word "ruined" or for that matter "malformed." The original rejection of the use of thalidomide by this country, the additional two years it had been kept on the shelf, and the concerns about its neurological toxicity that restricted its distribution are all factors that saved American children from the same disaster that condemned European infants to a lifetime of being crippled.

The delay really only bought time, but that was enough, for during the two years that the use of thalidomide was restricted in the United States, two German physicians, seeing a growing number of infants being born without arms and legs, made the association between these deformities and the fact that the mothers of these congenitally malformed children had taken thalidomide during the first few months of their pregnancy. Why these two doctors and no one else made the connection is hard to determine. Perhaps they knew more or sensed more or were simply not willing to dismiss these deformed children as mistakes of nature or examples of a new, though still unexplainable type of fetal infection. Perhaps they simply talked to the mothers, or unlike other doctors, refusing to believe the placenta was a medical barrier, were the ones who asked these women if they had taken any drugs during their pregnancies or been exposed to any unique environmental poisons. Possibly they just cared more, were obsessed by the suffering of these poor children and their parents, and so were not willing, if anything could be done, to let others be born crippled too.

Whatever, at the time these two physicians made the association, the idea of drugs crossing the placenta was still not a generally accepted medical doctrine, yet they persisted in their investigation and soon, as more and more European infants were delivered without limbs, other physicians no longer able to ignore the increasing numbers of crippled children being born began making the same connection between the defects and the maternal use of thalidomide. Again it was a matter of the time lag. Even as the German doctors were discovering they were right, other pregnant women continued to be given the drug while those who had already taken it but had not yet delivered could do nothing but wait and see what would be born to them.

It was soon discovered, once studies of the drug were undertaken, that as many as 40 percent of the women who had taken the drug during the first three months of their pregnancies had delivered children with the limb deformities. Forty percent from a drug that the American distributor, the Merrell company, was later to state it had had every reason to believe harmless and fit for human use!

Even more frightening than Merrell's denouncement of its own culpability or even the crippled children themselves was the realization that had the defects caused by thalidomide been any less dramatic or less noticeable—such as minimal brain damage, partial blindness, severe far-sightedness or motor dysfunction—or had the deformities been similar to those already known to be due to naturally occurring genetic defects or chromosomal abnormalities such as dislocated hips or harelips, no one would have noticed for years that the increase in these defects was due to the ingestion of a drug. The drug might well have been used to ruin a whole generation, perhaps more. It was only the catastrophic dimensions of the injury, the dramatic nature of the defect that alerted physicians to what we were doing to ourselves.

With the report of the association of thalidomide with fetal limb-bud abnormalities, the Merrell pharmaceutical house, unlike the drug companies of Europe, was given the chance to cut its losses and get out. It is unpleasant to speculate on disasters, but medical experts are of the opinion that with our high level of drug dependence, the supposed low risk from the medication, and the large number of drugs prescribed for pregnant women, the drug, had it been released for general use in the United States, would have caused a major catastrophe. The number of American children born crippled would have been gigantic. It has been proposed that almost every family in America would in some way have been affected.

In August of 1962, prompted by the German report of thalidomide-associated congenital defects, Merrell sent out a letter to every physician in North America recalling each thalidomide pill that had been manufactured and either distributed in Canada as a prescription drug or released in the United States as part of the clinical trial.

The letter, dated August 10, 1962, is still filed away in pediatricians' offices across the country. It began simply enough. "To all Physicians. Last November came the first reports of a sharply rising incidence of phocomelia in some European countries and the possible association of the drug, thalidomide, with it. We at Merrell were deeply and sympathetically concerned. At that time thalidomide, under the Merrell label, was on prescription sold in Canada, and undergoing clinical evaluation in the United States. Recently this tragedy of congenital malformation has received wide publicity. . . ."

The letter went on to state: "Prior to the first reports of

congenital malformation Merrell and its investigation had every reason to believe that thalidomide was a highly useful and non-toxic substitute for barbiturates." No such letter could be sent to the parents of the thousands of deformed children in Europe. Years later a lawsuit against Distillers Ltd., the distributors of thalidomide in England, would cost that company $64 million in damages, approximately $20,000 per arm and leg that had never grown and never would, $40,000 per child who would never be able to run or hold out his own arms.

Merrell's recall letter was truthful in stating that prior to the first reports of thalidomide-induced congenital malformations, the drug was indeed considered safe, that indeed there was no reason to believe that if given to pregnant women it would turn what should have been a blessing and a joy into a lifetime of tragedy and heartache. But what was also true, though not mentioned in the letter, was the fact that the drug had never been adequately tested for safety in pregnant women. The concept of placental transfer of drugs, if not a generally accepted medical doctrine at the time of the North American distribution of thalidomide, was certainly well enough established for the manufacturers of drugs to at least be concerned about it; yet thalidomide was released to the general population as if no one had ever heard of the concept.

The millions of dollars awarded to the parents of the English children in what was eventually called the "Thalidomide Tragedy" were given not out of the good will of the courts of England, but because the British justices would not accept for Distillers Ltd. the concept of nonresponsibility that lay behind Merrell's recall letter. It was the judgment of the British court that Distillers was responsible. To the court there were obviously some things so self-evident that no other side could be accepted, no other argument presented. The lack of arms and legs spoke for itself.

4.

What really happened in the case of thalidomide was well beyond courts and lawsuits, beyond suffering and grief, beyond even culpability or innocence. What happened was chemistry, unconcerned and unfeeling, a province older than life itself.

Between the eighth and tenth weeks of human fetal development the embryonic cells that will eventually give rise to the newly forming baby's arms and legs, begin to take shape as observable little outpocketings along the sides of the embryo. It is during this time of embryonic life and only this time that the limb-bud cells, programmed from the beginning to form the limbs, begin to separate themselves out from all the rest of the embryo's cells. Those few cells will eventually form all the finished bones and blood vessels, the muscles and nerves of the infant's arms and legs.

What scientists studying the "Thalidomide Tragedy" later discovered was to become one of the most disturbing facts to confront physicians concerned with preventive medicine in perhaps the whole last half-century. The scientists discovered that in many cases it took only one thalidomide pill, one trip to the medicine cabinet, one night of trying to get to sleep, one pill borrowed from a friend or taken by mistake—less than 5/1000 of a gram—to ruin a child for life, to put an end to any development or hope of development of its arms or legs. The drug was discovered, to everyone's astonishment, to be invariably effective in producing deformities in human embryos. The original estimates of 40 percent of pregnant women who had taken the drug giving birth to defective infants had to be revised upward. The incidence of malformations was found to be, if the drug had been taken at exactly the time the limb buds were beginning to form, closer to 100 percent.

As the fetal limb-bud cells began to differentiate themselves from all the other developing cells of the embryo's body, they became susceptible to thalidomide. In some physical or chemical way the configuration of the internal compounds developing inside those few differentiating limb buds, the unique combinations of their own internal carbons and hydrogen atoms just the shape of the compounds and enzymes being internally assembled by these cells' genetic material to take them on to the next step of fetal development, matched the chemistry of the molecules of thalidomide that had entered the fetal circulation. The unique intracellular compounds produced by these limb-bud cells at the very beginning of their development were destroyed, and the limb-bud cells containing them either died or were so injured by the destruction that they could not continue to differentiate. We do not need our arms or legs to live, so the embryo minus its few limb-bud cells continued to grow, its other fetal cells going on unconcerned to form the heart and lungs, the brain and liver, developing on as if nothing had occurred.

What happened if a pregnant woman took thalidomide during that crucial period of her child's limb-bud development was as simple as it was terrible. After she swallowed the pill, its outer coating dissolved in the hydrochloric acid of her stomach and the chemical liberated was absorbed into her bloodstream, where it was carried by her circulation to all the parts of her body. The drug not only entered her own brain cells, interfering with their own intracellular structures making her sleepy, but also crossed the placenta and entered her child's circulation, where it was carried throughout his developing body as well.

If she swallowed the pill at any other time than when the limb-bud cells were beginning to be formed, the drug, taken up by virtually all the embryo's fetal cells, simply lay around in them, an inert intruder, until it was metabolized, destroyed, or moving back out of the cells into the bloodstream, circulated back to the mother, where it was excreted. But if she took the thalidomide during those critical seven to fourteen days when the limb buds of her child were just beginning to differentiate, the drug, getting into those early cells and coupling with their intracellular enzymes, either destroyed the cells or injured them so severely that they stopped developing totally or their development was so slowed down that under the strict time scheme and economy of fetal development, their time for interaction with the other cells of the embryo passed and with it the one chance for the fetus to develop its arms and legs.

For all the assertiveness of life and its seeming dominion, its continuation and maintenance are still a very close affair. It is that very closeness which haunts knowledgeable researchers today, and worries physicians, but especially pediatricians who understand that a mistake occurring early in the life of any child can be a mistake forever.

5.

Embryologists learned early that they could reproductively produce a defect, the same defect, in newborn animals by injuring each developing fetus in exactly the same way. Researchers working with sheep embryos, removing the fetus early in its development, keeping its maternal blood supply intact, have been able to put the embryo under the dissecting microscope. By removing or destroying a few of the millions of developing cells, then putting the fetus back in the uterus to continue its development, they were able—depending on the time after fertilization when they injured the fetal cells, the type of injury produced and the method used, as well as the cell type destroyed—to produce different kinds of congenital defects, defects easily seen in the animals after they were born.

Except for the removal or injury of those few dividing embryonic cells, the fetus had not been injured or damaged in any way, yet depending on which cells were removed or damaged and at what time of gestation the injury occurred, totally different and at times devastating congenital defects could be reproductively produced in animal after animal. By destroying or removing similar cells from different sheep embryos at the same stage of their embryologic development, the researchers could produce the exact same congenital defect in each of the newborn animals—the same brain defect, the same congenital heart, the same defective lung. They could produce embryos born blind or deaf, fetuses with no jaw or no legs. They could, by finding and injuring or destroying the right cell or group of cells, have the animals born hypothyroid or with no thyroid at all.

What these researchers proved is what the first embryologists had thought for years: that while each embryo is a totally new creature, the process of its unfolding is precisely regimented and completely ordered. The mechanics of embryonic development, cellular differentiation and intracellular interactions, immutable from fetus to fetus, are run by processes as exacting and as controlled as any physical process anywhere in nature. Each embryonic cell is a crucial part of the whole process, earmarked from its very beginning to form a certain part of the body, so that if even one cell is destroyed or damaged, the tissue or the organ that would normally develop from it is gone and gone forever.

The researchers found what they would have expected, since the first few fetal cells dividing from the fertilized egg give rise, through their own dividing, to all the other embryonic cells which come after; the earlier in gestation a fetal cell was injured, the more devastating were the effects on the fetus. Kill one fertilized egg itself, and no embryo would develop at all. Injure the earliest cells formed soon after conception and you would get some fetal development, but eventually the embryo would soon die and be resorbed; damage the fetal cells later in embryonic development and some organs would form but not others. Kill fetal cells still later when the embryos were well established, and the various organs themselves would develop but would be defective. Cause cellular injury early in fetal development and the fetus dies; injure its cells later and you get congenital defects.

But it is not even necessary to actually remove an embryo from its mother to injure fetal cells. It can all be done without touching the fetus at all. What happened with thalidomide was shown to have happened with anticonvulsants. Recently researchers found that they could routinely cause rats to be born with cleft palates by simply feeding their mothers a drug called Dilantin, a chemical used in humans as a medication for seizure disorders. It is possible by breeding rats to know exactly to the day when the females become pregnant. By using these timed pregnancies, and putting the drug in the rats' food at specific times following conception and at only those times, baby rats would be born with cleft lips and cleft palates.

Physically untouched, supposedly safely protected within their mothers, these embryos were as systematically ruined by what their mothers were eating as the sheep embryos had been by physical manipulations. Dilantin, like Dicumarol and radioactive iodine, crosses the placenta and like those other drugs interferes with a billion years of evolutionary control and chemical order, its unique chemical structure destroying, out of the millions of developing cells, only those few specific fetal cells that will be necessary for the normal development of the face, coupling with these cells and poisoning their intracellular chemicals so that the baby rats when born will have the roof of their mouths left open and their lips cleft down to the bone.

. . .

In 1968 S. R. Meadows, a physician at Guys Hospital in London, wrote in a typically restrained English manner a letter that was published in total by the medical journal *The Lancet.*

"I should be interested to know," the writer stated, "if your readers have seen babies with harelips, cleft palate, and certain other specific abnormalities born to mothers who received regular anticonvulsant therapy.

"Three years ago after encountering three such infants I contacted forty-eight mothers in the Brighton area who had children with harelips and cleft palates. None (of the mothers) had epilepsy, and only one had had an anticonvulsant during pregnancy. However, recently I have seen two more babies, born to epileptic mothers."

He went on to ask if any other doctors had noticed this association. They had. Two German physicians answered that they had found five babies with malformation among 225 babies born to epileptic mothers; three of these had cleft lips, without cleft palates.

The Dutch, prompted by Meadows' letter in *The Lancet,* began to look at their own children born to epileptic mothers who had received Dilantin during their pregnancies. They found that the rate of facial malformations in children born to these women was five times the rate in children born to nonepileptic mothers. Since it was possible that the cause of this increase in facial deformities might not be the drugs these women were taking but perhaps their disease itself, the Dutch physicians started their own meticulous experiments.

These were the first fetal animal toxicity studies done on anticonvulsants. Unfortunately, they were begun too late for those children already born with their deformed faces, but they did prove once and for all that just adding chemicals to the food of pregnant animals could injure fetal cells and cause

congenital defects. These studies showed that there were two
periods of embryonic development, day 9 and days 11 to 14,
when fetal rats were susceptible to Dilantin-induced facial
deformities. Other fetal soft tissues were affected as well. The
studies also proved what thalidomide had shown—the exquis-
ite time-relationship of the taking of drugs with the development of fetal defects.

Twenty-six random albino rats were used. All were injected
with 2.5 mg of Dilantin; 1.9 mg and 1.75 mg daily for a period
of four days at various times after mating. The mice had 233
offspring. In mice injected on day 10 following mating, no mice
were born—all were killed by the drug; the resorption was 100
percent, the mothers resorbing all the dead fetuses. Obviously,
on day 10 the newly developing embryonic cells were so susceptible to the drug, so many were injured or destroyed that none
were left to form any tissues, and all the embryos died. In those
injected with 1.75 mg just one day later—day 11—the resorption rate was only 15 percent and the mice born appeared
normal; the fetal cells in one day had changed enough to
become resistant to the drug. Yet at a dose of 1.9 mg, just two
tenths of a milligram more than the 1.75 mg that had apparently proved harmless in the fetuses not resorbed, over 15
percent of the embryos were born with cleft palates.

The production of cleft lips and palates was not only time-
related but dose-related. No one could ever again argue that
drugs given to pregnant women might not be damaging to
their fetuses. In truth, as the Dutch realized, all that spared
many more mothers the fate of seeing their children born with
deformed faces was the fact that epilepsy is a relatively rare
disease. If Dilantin had been as widely used as thalidomide, it
would have been deformed faces rather than no arms or legs
that would have shocked the world.

6.

We are now aware that drugs used during pregnancy can and do cause gross physical congenital defects. Yet the deeper concern is not with the gross defects caused by chemicals but the subtler and more difficult-to-evaluate effects of drugs on a developing child's personality, his intelligence and mental abilities as well as his motor coordination and psychological growth. If drugs can cause arms not to grow and faces to be left open, then they can certainly get into fetal brain cells leading to poor electrical transmissions or storage ability, interfering or coupling with subcellular structures, not enough to kill the cells but to affect their functioning, leading to seizures, hyperactivity and decreased intelligence. Yet a study done in 1960, before the thalidomide and Dilantin tragedies, and a similar analysis done less than three years ago, showed no major differences in the number of drugs prescribed for pregnant women.

The 1960 study of upper-middle-class American women indicated that the average pregnant woman took between 3 and 29 different drugs during the course of her pregnancy. The average number was 10.3 per woman. Another study at the time, conducted by the National Institutes of Health on 50,-000 pregnancies, revealed that over 900 different pharmaceuticals were used by American mothers during the course of their pregnancies. The simple fact is that the number of drugs being prescribed for pregnant women in 1972 hadn't changed. Bronchodilators, antihistamines, analgesics, barbiturates, antacids, antiemetics, water pills, iron pills, vitamins, cough medicines, hormones, tranquilizers, appetite suppressants, hypnotics, sulfonamides, penicillins, erythromycin, as well as dozens of other over-the-counter medications that women take themselves, are being used as freely today as in the early sixties.

The drug companies and the myth of the doctor as prescriber rather than healer have continued to triumph over common sense and reason. A recent government study showed that the average pregnant woman giving birth today is still taking in excess of ten medications, with at least four of these being prescribed by a physician.

If one evaluates the reaction of the medical profession to the thalidomide experience solely on the basis of the continuing use of drugs prescribed to pregnant women, it would appear that those thousands of thalidomide babies have had no effect on the medical profession or on society itself. Drugs are still being prescribed that have not been adequately tested.

In an article published in 1975 in the *Journal of Clinical Research* titled "Drug Therapy and the Developing Human— Who Cares," the author, a noted pharmacologist and pediatrician, felt compelled, because of his own specific concern for the emotional and intellectual health of children, to write about one type of drug—the most widely prescribed in America— tranquilizers. "The potential relationship between administration of psychoactive drugs [tranquilizers] to pregnant women and the development of abnormal or emotional patterns in their offspring has been discussed at scientific meetings. While there is currently little data to support such a contention, this question clearly needs resolution since one study in the United States reported 32 percent of all pregnant women surveyed were receiving tranquilizers."

The issue, though, of environmental poisons is not restricted to embryonic development. The reasons why fetal arms and legs don't grow and embryonic thyroids are destroyed, why faces don't form correctly and newborns bleed to death are the same reasons why tissues turn cancerous.

VI

The New Plague

1.

If there is any one overiding concern that haunts physicians today, one great fear that drives cancer researchers and keeps them working and publishing their findings in the face of powerful industrial and at times political opposition, not to mention personal and professional abuse, it is that a low-grade but potent cancer-causing substance may be introduced into the general environment unknowingly or uncaringly, to be consumed by vast numbers of people, dooming them before they even know about the inevitable and untreatable malignancies.

These researchers know that minute exposures of cells to carcinogenic compounds can lead to cancer, and that because of the uniqueness of malignant diseases, the long time lags between exposure and the development of overt cancers—in humans as long as twenty-five to thirty years—a carcinogen, if distributed among the general population, might well doom hundreds of thousands, perhaps even millions of people before the harmful effects of the chemical become obvious enough to

stop any further distribution. Whole generations could be
wasted before we would even know we were in danger. The
dead would be our first warning and the dying would continue
for decades until those last to be exposed would themselves
finally be buried.

The grim fact is that this has already happened. The researchers' greatest fear has already come true.

Beginning in 1941, in the name of patriotism, with the tacit
agreement of the federal government and the wholehearted
cooperation of the American Red Cross, almost every healthy
young adult male between the ages of eighteen and twenty-six
in the entire U.S. population was systematically if unknowingly
exposed to a low-grade but potent carcinogenic. From Guadal-
canal on, the exposure was massive and continual. The USO,
religious groups, friends and relatives, all made sure their young
men, no matter where they were, received cartons of cigarettes.
What from World War I had grown into an individual habit
became with World War II a national institution.

It is not far-fetched today to say that the cigarettes delivered
month after month to the Marines on Guam and Saipan, the
airmen flying out of Tinian and Iceland, the Third Army
pushing up through the Rhine Valley, the 101st and 82nd
Airborne in Holland and Belgium, would eventually prove as
deadly to those young men as any German bullet or Japanese
rocket. Those cigarettes would eventually kill as many of them
as any grenade or mine.

The dying from coal tars began well before World War II.
Earle, Bennet, Von Volkmann, all pointed out the dangers well
over a hundred and fifty years ago. Like Sir Percivall Pott, they
were surgeons who proved that the cancers they saw in their
patients were due to exposure to industrial compounds. Their
studies had nothing to do with rats or rabbits, but with people.
Theirs were already the ultimate experiments.

Pott showed that the terrible skin cancers occurring in the groins of chimney sweeps were due to the fact that their skin had been continually exposed to the soot lining the chimney walls and gratings in which they worked. In a series of brilliant studies he proved that the reason these cancers were restricted to the scrotal skin of the workers and no other areas of their bodies was that the soot they were exposed to accumulated in their pants and that while they washed their hands and faces after work, they were not as careful about their groins; the coal tars stayed there, becoming embedded in the skin folds.

He found cancers in sweeps whose ages ran from eighteen to forty-seven, and while he couldn't explain the reason for the age spread, he did call attention to the fact that the younger chimney sweeps who developed skin cancer were those who had begun working in the chimneys when they were three and four years of age; the older chimney sweeps with cancers had started their exposures later in life.

Surgeons all over the world found similar occurrences in other petroleum-based industries: the tar and paraffin workers of Hale, the workers in the Lancashire cotton and spinning mills, the men who lubricated the industries' machines in Cardiff. All developed cancers, and all had the same long latency period discovered in the chimney sweeps, and later to be observed in the Japanese animal studies. For the last hundred years there has been ample and abundant evidence that cancer of the skin can be caused by industrial exposures to soot, coal tar, pitch and mineral oils, all of which are compounds containing the same chemicals present in cigarette smoke.

By the 1900's the stage was set. The first scientific facts about the dangers of coal tars were in, but the real drama began in the 1910's, when for the first time a very small but select group of international accountants, the vital statisticians, noted an increase in the incidence of lung cancer. It was their data, the result of tabulating the death rates in various countries, that became the starting point for the first studies on the relationship between the uses of tobacco and lung cancer, as well as diseases of the heart and the respiratory system.

For thirty years these vital statisticians chronicled the deaths of a whole generation, writing their reports in obscure journals, filling endless columns with rows of cold emotionless numbers denoting the ever increasing incidence of human deaths from lung cancer.

In 1928 Lombard and Doering, trying to explain this increase in lung cancer, published an article in the *New England Journal of Medicine* entitled "Cancer Studies in Massachusetts and Habits, Characteristics and Environment of Individuals with and without Cancer." They showed, among other things, an association between heavy smoking and cancer.

In 1939 Miller, a German physician who had noticed over the twenty years of his own practice, beginning in 1918, an increasing percentage of lung cancer diagnosed at autopsy examinations in and around his city of Cologne, devised the first study to explore this association, to see if there was indeed a connection between cigarette smoking and the increased incidence of cancer. Very early in his study it became clear that this increased incidence was occurring almost exclusively in men. After considering other possible causes for the increase —street dust, automobile exhaust, poison-gas exposure in World War I, increased use of X-rays, influenza, trauma, tuberculosis and waste exposure due to industrial growth—he attributed the increased incidence of lung cancer to the increase in tobacco consumption that had begun in Germany shortly before World War I. After carefully inquiring of family and friends into the smoking habits of his lung-cancer victims, he published the first conclusive data showing that there was an excess of heavy smokers among those men who had died of malignancies of the lung.

It was during this time that the active cancer-causing material in both coal tars and industrial oils was isolated and found to be benzopyrene, the most potent cancer-causing ingredient ever discovered.

It was also during this time that Peyton Rous made his discovery, setting the stage for Berenblum's work. It was Berenblum, though, who, a few years after Miller's publication, having established that once a cell was rendered premalignant due to exposure to a carcinogen, it stayed that way, never reverting back to normal, made the definitive statement concerning cancer. "Cells may become neoplastic [cancerous] in considerable numbers," he wrote, "yet never manifest themselves unless ordered by extraneous influences [irritation]. When one considers this finding in the light of the proven abilities of human cancer cells to persist for years without asserting themselves it becomes plain that the trauma which is followed by the prompt appearance of a tumor in tissue that has previously appeared normal may act merely by stimulating neoplastic elements already long present. A carcinogenic agent may do its work years before and the cells it renders neoplastic have remained ever since within their morphological context, incapable of asserting themselves until some intercurrent accident, a blow, a wound, or burn [irritation] stirs them to proliferate."

A clearer warning could not have been given. Like the clicking of a terrible grandfather's clock, those words written in the nineteen-forties echo today down our thousands of sterile cancer wards, past the beds of men and women, our aunts and uncles, our sisters and brothers, all dying decades before their time.

2.

Within a few years after the end of World War II, the increasing incidence of lung cancers was no longer restricted to the awareness of a few concerned physicians and worried statisticians. By 1950 almost every surgeon in America was beginning to notice the increase among his male patients. All across the nation, in doctors' offices, in clinics, in outpatient departments and hospital emergency rooms, more and more men were being shown their X-rays and told they would soon be dead. By the nineteen-fifties the incidence of malignancies of the lung had risen from the 4 per 100,000 of the population of the twenties to well over 25 per 100,000, the major increase occurring in the years following World War II.

This startling increase was said at first to signify only an apparent increase, the result of the better diagnostic techniques that had only recently then come into routine medical use, the increased use of chest X-rays as well as utilization of the new clinical skills which medicine had acquired and learned to use both during and after the war. Physicians ignoring or refusing to accept the work of Rous and Berenblum, Miller and Lombard, complimented themselves on their new abilities, declaring that lung cancers had always been there in such numbers, only now they were finally being detected. Some physicians even intimated that on the average they were better doctors than had been available to previous generations, that if nothing else their newly developed machines, monitoring apparatus and laboratory facilities gave them the edge in diagnosis.

But by 1955 no one would be saying that any more. The incidence of lung cancer continued to increase so greatly— doubling again by the middle fifties—that by 1956 no one could attribute the growth to anything other than a sudden actual increase in the disease itself.

As concerned physicians continued to watch, the incidence went straight up off the charts. By 1960 it was 40 per 100,000, by 1965 it was 50. Coughing and wheezing, men in greater and greater numbers were going to their doctors expecting to be told they had congestion and instead were told they had lung cancer.

In 1933 Cook had isolated benzopyrene from coal tars. In the late forties it was identified as a component of cigarette smoke. More recent techniques have defined the chemistry of smoking even further. A recent article put it simply: "Benzopyrene is one of the two most potent of the seven carcinogens detected in cigarette smoke and it is present in much larger quantity than any of the other carcinogens." The carcinogens were there, and as with Pott's chimney sweeps and Rous's rabbits, continued to do their work.

By the mid-fifties, twenty-nine separate retrospective studies of lung cancer had been compiled, all indicating a relationship between the development of the cancer and cigarette smoking. Physicians at the National Cancer Institute, members of the American Cancer Society and the American Heart Association, unable to ignore this gathering of data, the growing number of men dying each year, decided to act.

They were met with almost instant opposition. Following the publication of several important retrospective studies in the years 1952–1956, the presidents of these prestigious organizations asked the Surgeon General and the U.S. Public Health Service to become officially engaged in the appraisal of all the available data on the relationship between cigarette smoking and health.

In June 1956 a scientific study group was established jointly by the National Cancer Institute, the National Heart Institute, the American Cancer Society and the American Heart Association. After evaluating sixteen independent studies that had gone on in five separate countries over the preceding eighteen years, the group in late 1956 concluded there was definitely a relationship between smoking and lung cancer. On July 12, 1957, the Surgeon General issued a statement based on the report of the study group: "The Public Health Service feels the weight of the evidence is increasingly pointing in one direction: That excessive smoking is one of the correlative factors in lung cancer."

The statement was made and there it rested. The deaths went on. The cigarette advertisements continued to show lovely mountain streams and handsome people riding their horses along beautiful seashores. The truth was less idyllic but much more dramatic: vigorous men bleeding to death and having to gasp for air as they slowly and painfully wasted away.

Two years later the Surgeon General, faced with the continually increasing incidence of lung-cancer deaths among Americans, issued a more forceful statement: "Cigarette smoking particularly is associated with an increased chance of developing cancer." Still nothing was done and physicians across the country continued to watch their patients die, and the deaths were not the clean simple affairs seen on television dramatizations, but brutal terrifying events.

A recent study has shown that 36 percent of cancer patients do not die from their cancers but from the uncontrolled infections that complicate their malignancies. There are days of fever and vomiting, headaches and chills; then the blood pressure falls, hearts dilate and lungs fill with fluid. Eighteen percent simply hemorrhage to death. Perhaps they die at home, or in the park, or walking to their cars; they die in the open with no one to help; they die at picnics and football games. Vomiting blood, they bleed to death while their relatives and neighbors just stand there watching helplessly, unable to do a thing. Five percent die more slowly, more painfully, from liver failures; 19 percent by breathing in their own vomit. Seven percent die from their hearts giving out. One percent just waste away. The rest simply die.

And it doesn't end with the deaths. Almost 80 percent of all families of cancer patients admit to having had, within their families, during or shortly after the illness, severe emotional problems, difficult psychological adjustment reactions. Wives confess to feelings of guilt and resentment against their dying husbands. Children watching their fathers die become confused and agitated, refuse to go to school or to listen, while other children, left to themselves when their mothers go to the hospital and angered at being left alone, become delinquent or run away. Cancer deaths, too, take time. Homes have to be sold to pay the bills, life savings are depleted, vacations abandoned. Everyone in some way is affected. Smoking is depicted by tobacco companies as something sophisticated and worldly, but it is not the sophistication and worldliness expressed by one wife when she said, "In the end, you just want him to die and get it over with."

3.

On June 1, 1961, a letter urging the formation of a presidential commission to study the "widespread implications of the tobacco problem" was sent to the President of the United States and signed by the presidents of the American Cancer Society, the American Public Health Association, the American Heart Association and the National Tuberculosis Association.

On July 27, 1962, a list of more than a hundred and fifty physicians and scientists working in the fields of biology and medicine were compiled as potential members for what was to become the Surgeon General's Advisory Committee. From that list, ten men were selected who agreed to serve on the committee and were named "The Surgeon General's Advisory Committee on Smoking and Health."

The lines were finally drawn. Death hung in the balance and it was death that won. Greed, corruption and avarice have held the day. Common sense, compassion, concern and humanity are ignored.

From the issuing of the first reports in the early fifties on the relationship between cancer and smoking, the tobacco industry took to defending itself against any responsibility for the increase by simply ignoring the figures and stating that the disease was really nothing new, that it had always been a human problem. That was true, but by 1961 the problem was not the presence of lung cancer, but the numbers.

The committee, in going over all the available data, all the studies and reports, agreed with the tobacco industry that lung cancer had always been a human problem. There had always been a certain low but constant level of malignancies of the lung, just as there had always been a small but consistent incidence of spontaneous brain tumors and kidney cancers. But beginning with the moderate increase in smoking during World War I and following the gigantic increase in consumption of cigarettes during World War II, the incidence had soared. Moreover, while the cancers had formerly occurred in older people, they were now appearing in younger and younger men. The issue was not that there was a new kind of cancer in the world, but that there was more of the old one and that the old one was occurring in men at younger ages.

But the numbers were only part of the problem. What troubled the committee as much as the increasing incidence of lung cancer was the fact that there appeared to be no adequate treatment. Even with the removal of the tumor, even with radiation and chemotherapy, the one-year survivals were virtually zero. The diagnosis of lung cancer was essentially a death sentence. The committee was sitting in the midst of an epidemic that was proving more deadly than polio or smallpox.

By the mid-sixties it was clear that malignant transformations were caused by some kind of subcellular injury, that carcinogenic compounds like the chemicals that poisoned fetal cells leading to congenital malformations cause cancer by getting into mature cells and injuring or poisoning intracellular enzymes and structures so that the cell lost its own internal controls.

Cancer is anarchy at a cellular level. Normal cells turned malignant are like soldiers with head wounds who suddenly go berserk. All this was known by the time the Advisory Committee was empaneled; the real question was not that malignant transformations occurred but exactly what it was that disrupted the internal machinery so that cells took off on their own.

One of the theories proposed at the time the committee was selected was that the cause was genetic, that cells turn malignant because their genes tell them to. The idea was that a gene sitting in the cell's nucleus, one that had been suppressed for years, even decades, suddenly expressed itself and and the cell under new nuclear control took off on a new and destructive path. Another theory maintained that the malignant cell was changed by a virus, one that had gotten into the cell and by growing there, disrupted the delicate internal control mechanisms just by being there, causing the cell to become cancerous. Another theory attributed malignant changes to nothing more than normal cellular wear and tear, a subcellular breakdown similar to a car suddenly going out of control because of a simple wearing out of an overused piece of metal. Still another claimed defects in the immune response system—continuing antigenic stimulation, overloading cellular function or a lack of immune surveillance—as the cause of malignant transformations.

Diverse as these theories seem on the surface, they all contained at their core the same fundamental proposition: cancer develops in once normal cells that have somehow been changed internally. Where the theories differed was in their explanation of what caused the change.

The Surgeon General's Advisory Committee quickly disposed of genetics as a possible cause of the increase in lung cancer. Although both men and women have essentially the same genetic information in their cells, the increase in the disease was due almost entirely to the numbers of men affected. Virus as a potential cause was also quickly eliminated. If the epidemic of lung cancer was being caused by a virus, it would have to be a strange virus indeed that affected only men, and again, only men in their late forties, fifties and sixties. Viruses infect both men and women alike; they have never showed any sexual preference in human epidemics or in animal studies.

It was possible that the increasing incidence of lung cancer could have been due to a gradually wearing out of subcellular control mechanisms, but again, why only men and not women? The well-documented weakening of the immune system in older people might have been the cause. Yet the patients evaluated by the committee were not older men, and again, the natural decay of immunity occurs equally in men and women. If antigenic stimulation, cellular breakdown or the lack of immune surveillance was what led to these cancers, then the increased incidence should have been equal among men and women, but it wasn't.

This left only one cause: an environmental carcinogen, something that men were exposed to and not women; a cellular poison that was unique since not only did it not seem to affect women, but it did not bother children either, nor for that matter, any other living thing; only men between forty and sixty years of age.

The committee began its retrospective studies by going over

the case histories of those who had already died from lung cancer, comparing their histories with the histories of matched controls—people of the same age, socioeconomic background and religious preferences—who had not died from lung cancers. Using computers and calculators to help analyze the data, the committee found that the only difference between those men dying of lung cancer and those who were not was cigarettes. There was no other difference. The vast majority of those who had died of the disease had smoked cigarettes, while virtually no one acquired the disease who did not smoke.

The committee's first report was finally published in 1964 under the title "Smoking and Health: Report of the Advisory Committee to the Surgeon General of the Public Health Service." It was met with instant anger and even derision by the tobacco industry. While tobacco lobbyists descended on Washington to buttonhole senators and congressmen, and company officials visited the various governmental regulation agencies, a flood of pro-smoking propaganda was released to the media and pressed into advertising campaigns.

In that first confrontation the tobacco apologists had one good point to argue and they hammered away at it: the type of studies the committee had relied on. Indeed, it is the one valid criticism of the report, a criticism that in truth can never be answered because it deals with the intrinsic weakness of any retrospective study. A retrospective study is one that depends on data collected from past records, personal histories, medical and mortality records of individuals studied as members of a group. It is a study that is done after the fact, and there are always limitations and the possibility of errors in the types of questions set up to distinguish between groups.

What the committee did was go over the medical and social histories of people who had already died from lung cancer and question relatives about the habits and activities of the victims, then compare these results with a similar evaluation of a control group. The committee asked many questions, one of which was about smoking habits, and found that the one thing that separated the two groups was the question of whether they smoked or not.

The tobacco industry immediately challenged the committee's findings. Maybe it wasn't the smoking; maybe it was coffee, or tea. What happened if the smokers were also deep breathers and took in more polluted air than nonsmokers? What the tobacco industry was complaining about was that the committee had not checked everything, every possible relationship between the lung-cancer patients and the matched controls, so how could they be sure it was cigarette smoking that was at fault and not something else?

The industry was right in that retrospective studies only give correlations between questions that are asked, not those that aren't. But the members of the committee were not fools. They had not picked possible relationships at random merely to fill up computer time, or to be able to write a report. They were trying to find out why men were dying.

They looked at the relationship between lung cancer and cigarette smoking rather than coffee drinking or tooth brushing because it was the lungs of these men that had turned cancerous, not their stomachs or their mouths, and it was not the deeper parts of the lungs that were turning malignant but the cells lining the tubes that carried the air down from the mouth. The committee reasoned that if it was the cells lining these airways that were affected, and everyone was breathing essentially the same air, then there had to be something different in the air breathed by those who had developed lung cancer. They set up their study to ask, among other things, about possible inhaled carcinogens, and cigarette smoking was obviously something to ask about. They had no idea what the

results would show, but it was plain that cigarette smoking had
to be considered. It was checked out and the computers said
yes.

4.

The attack on the retrospective nature of the Surgeon General's report was pressed. But the tobacco industry realized that
they had a shaky case in rejecting all of the 387 pages of the
1964 report solely on the grounds of its retrospective nature,
so they began hammering away at the statistics—not just the
statistics of the report itself, but statistics in general. There was
no definitive proof that smoking caused cancer, they insisted,
just statistics. It was in the years that the tobacco companies
began attacking the statistical nature of the Surgeon General's
report that adults who had started to smoke after the end of
World War II began coughing up blood.

Perhaps in the airy realm of probabilities and percentages,
the tobacco-industry executives and their public relations offic-
ers had some vague mathematical, if not ethical or moral
grounds on which to attack the statistics of the first Surgeon
General's report. Probabilities are just that—probabilities—
and percentages are only percentages. But in the real world
they are adequate examples of risk, and if you happen to become part of a statistic, for you it is no longer a matter of
probabilities.

The real problem with statistics has nothing to do with their
inability to define specific risks; for that they are profoundly
accurate and more reliable than any casual observation or even
simple sampling. The problem is that they aren't personal. We
want—indeed, as a nation we demand—to see the gun pointed
at us before we become frightened or even concerned.

Standard errors, means, variances, standard deviations may only be statistical tools, but in cases where we are hunting for hidden causes or relationships, risks we are not yet quite sure of, they are the only tools we have, the only means in a confusing world of possibilities of finding out exactly what the dangers are, where they are and how they work. For all the use of percentages, statistics are precision tools that become more accurate, more definitive, more precise as we narrow down the questions asked, as we learn to ask better questions.

The questions got better: How many cigarettes were smoked? For how long? When did the smoking begin? Did the deceased inhale deeply? But the tobacco companies continued to confuse the issue by attacking not the data the committee was compiling, but the means and standard errors that had made the findings possible.

Yet it was not in their attacks on the retrospective nature of the Surgeon General's report or even on the statistical nature of the data that the tobacco apologists were most effective in confusing the issues and subverting the truth, but rather in their manipulation of one of our nation's most biased ideas about disease; and in this the medical establishment itself, as well as the rest of us, has in a sense been their ally.

We all tend to think of illness in instantaneous terms. You get infected, run a fever, go to the doctor, get a shot, get better. Feel the pain in your stomach? Go to the surgeon, be operated on and walk out of the hospital as good as new. It is a very limited view both of the practice of medicine and of disease. Actually, it is a view that is barely thirty years old, one which began only with the discovery of antibiotics and which has been kept alive by the continuing development of the ever more complicated modern-day surgical procedures—heart transplants, lung resections, arterial grafts, coronary bypass, with all their stunning, if limited, achievements.

Physicians themselves have maintained this idea of instant disease because it gives them their value, what they think people consider important—treatment and cure. Get operated on, have your uterus out, have your gall bladder removed, feel fine again. No problem, no worry. People expect something for their money, and physicians consciously or unconsciously have given their effort to supporting the comforting idea that diseases are immediate and can be instantly treated and quickly cured. But this idea is applicable to an ever decreasing number of infectious diseases and an even greater shrinking number of specific surgical conditions.

Talk to anyone with arthritis or ulcerative colitis, people with degenerative bone diseases, sickle cell anemia or thalassemia, children with muscular dystrophy, chronic glomerulonephritis or cystic fibrosis, patients after their coronary bypass, or the people on dialysis, adults going blind from diabetes. Ask those suffering from chronic lung disease, recurrent urinary-tract infections, seizure disorders or mental retardation—ask them what they think of the idea that all illness begins quickly, is quickly diagnosed or diagnosable, and quickly cured. They know and their families know.

Except for certain infectious diseases and some operative conditions, the majority of human illnesses are, if not slowly progressive, at least chronic or recurrent. The idea of the instantaneousness of disease, as well as of rapid and simple cures, is nothing more than a cultural bias. But it is a powerful notion and the tobacco companies exploit it to the fullest. Within months of the publication of the Surgeon General's report on smoking, testimonials were being heard all across the country: "Hell, I know people who've smoked ten and twenty years, and they're okay" . . . "My grandfather smoked every day of his life and he's all right" . . . "My uncle smokes and he's never got into trouble."

But cancer is not a simple pneumonia or urinary-tract infection, nor is it an appendicitis attack. It has no more in common with a cold or meningitis than its treatment does with cough medicines or penicillin. Cancer is a totally different kind of disease. It has its own rules and its own relentless course. There is no one day of feeling bad, a day or two of fever or listlessness, a visit to the doctor, a diagnosis, a shot and everything is better. Cancer is different.

Malignancies do not develop overnight; experiment after experiment has shown that once cells are exposed to a carcinogen it takes years—in the case of humans, decades—before they undergo complete degeneration and become overtly malignant. Cancer is a different kind of disease, with its own unique rules.

5.

Within a few years after the committee report was published, the incidence of lung cancer in the United States had risen to almost 55 per 100,000—double the incidence that had itself prompted the study in the first place, and over ten times that noted before the mass exposure begun during World War II.

Yet the criticisms leveled by the tobacco companies against the retrospectiveness of the committee's report continued, as did their attack on the statistical nature of the evaluation. The public's view of disease and disease processes as exploited by the industry, as well as the concern of most people about the issue of "statistics," only gave weight to their methodological criticisms. Knowing how the tobacco industry had attacked the first reports of the mid-fifties, the ten experts who had originally been chosen for the Surgeon General's Advisory Committee anticipated the objections their own study would face.

Even before they published their 1964 report they began a number of prospective studies. If the tobacco industry, the government and the general population, even physicians, needed a body count, they would give it to them.

A prospective study is a study in which men and women still alive are chosen at random or from some specific group, such as a profession, organization, socioeconomic class or religious sect, and are then followed to see what happens to them from the time of their entry into the study for an indefinite period, in this case until they died or were lost from follow-up because of other events.

Such a study can be as simple as it is brutal. And it was. The committee selected groups of men of the same age, same socioeconomic class, same life style, divided the number into those who smoked and those who did not, and then just waited to see what happened. There was no confusion now as to whether these men smoked or drank coffee, how much they really smoked or how deeply they inhaled, no question as to the brand of cigarette or even if they breathed more deeply than their neighbors. All this could be determined first hand—from the men themselves. None of the arguments against retrospective studies would hold now.

Prudence, though, common sense, suggested that at the very least, while the prospective studies were being conducted, what had already been learned from the first Surgeon General's report should have been used if not to stop smoking, at least to slow down its use, at the very minimum to keep children and adolescents from beginning their own exposures. Time was really all the committee asked for, but the tobacco companies and their lobbyists would have none of it. Smoking continued. No laws were passed, there were no restrictions on usage.

The committee, immobilized by the industry, had no choice but to wait for the results of the prospective study, for the dead bodies to fill the blank columns of their charts. And while they waited more people, not just those already in the studies but new ones, mostly children and adolescents, were beginning to smoke, exposing another whole generation. While our fathers and our brothers, our uncles and our friends became the statistics for the prospective study—their newly dug graves replacing the maligned means and belittled standard errors of the retrospective studies—another generation was beginning its own destruction.

In 1967 the second Surgeon General's report containing the results of the prospective studies confirmed and strengthened the retrospective conclusions of the 1964 report. The opening sentences of the new report stated: "Additional evidence from four major prospective studies indicates that cigarette smokers have marked increased risk of dying. . . . Even relatively young cigarette smokers have demonstrable respiratory symptoms."

The prospective studies gave the specifics that no retrospective study could ever hope to give. Not only did they definitely prove that, all other things being equal, cigarettes caused or significantly influenced the production of lung cancer in smokers versus nonsmokers, but the production of the malignancy was related to the *amount* of smoking, the *duration* of smoking, and *the age* at which smoking began. "Mortality rates exhibit a consistent and rather striking increase as the age at which smoking starts decreases. For men who started smoking cigarettes under the age of twenty, the over-all death rate was about twice that for non-smokers, whereas for those who did not start until they were twenty-five, the death rate was only 35% higher."

The prospective studies showed even more. The relationship between smoking and lung cancer also held for cancer of the larynx. Pipe and cigar smokers were found to be less affected than were cigarette smokers, whose death rates compared to nonsmokers was highest at the earliest age (forty to fifty). The conclusion at the end of the second report was as ominous as the conclusion of the first: "Deaths from lung cancer in the U.S. are continuing to rise rapidly."

Even with the publication of the second report, nothing happened. Our cultural bias toward disease made a public understanding of cancer with its acceptance of the dangers of carcinogenic exposure almost impossible. The power of vested interests—the hundreds of millions of dollars spent yearly on cigarette advertising in newspapers and magazines, insurance companies owned wholly or partially by conglomerates whose incomes were partially derived from tobacco-related industries keeping premiums of smokers as low as nonsmokers—all the lobbying and all the propaganda held the day even against the new set of prospective body counts.

Since no one was paying attention, the committee decided to publish its population studies. If the findings of both the retrospective and prospective studies were correct—and the committee was sure they were—then there should have been very little or no lung cancer among nonsmokers in the population. Studies undertaken of groups who for religious or moral reasons did not smoke revealed the incidence of the disease among these people to be almost zero. People breathing the same air as their neighbors, drinking the same water, eating the same food, living the same kind of life but not smoking, did not develop lung cancer while neighbors living right next door but smoking were dying of it. As for the effects of air pollution and urbanization the most that could be said was that they had some minor influence on the mortality rate from the disease. The committee also published the astonishing data proving that the total tars in cigarette smoke had forty times the carcinogenic potency of benzopyrene itself.

The results of the prospective studies should by themselves, without the addition of any further data, have led the government to prohibit the manufacture and sale of cigarettes. Coupled with the retrospective studies and the special-population-group studies, they should have induced the people of this country, and those sworn to protect them, to think of cigarette smoking the way they had come to think of cholera and typhus.

Yet as the committee had expected, the tobacco industry went after the prospective and population studies just as they had attacked the retrospective study. Statistics, they said again, small numbers, just probabilities. Again the testimonials were trotted out, and again the government bowed to the pressures of industry. As for the public, all they got was a tiny warning on the corner of each pack of cigarettes that smoking "might" be hazardous to their health.

6.

That "might" was finally put to rest by a third study, neither retrospective nor prospective, a study that did not even deal with ultimate outcomes of smokers versus nonsmokers, that did not have to wait for comparisons of twenty- and thirty-year results, a study in which there were practically no means or standard errors, a study that did not deal with the results of malignancies but with the beginnings of cancer itself.

If cigarette smoking caused lung cancer and if the disease took years of exposure to develop, as each of the studies had indicated, and if those tumors came from already premalignant cells, as Berenblum had stated following his experimental studies, then there would have to be some evidence of these precancerous transformations in the lungs of moderate smokers or those who had just begun to smoke. To definitively prove the environmental nature of lung cancer and its relationship to smoking, to demonstrate that lung cancers had nothing to do with infections, genetics or immunosuppression, to silence once and for all the tobacco industry and its supporters, precancerous lesions would have to be found in human lungs exposed to cigarette smoke for shorter periods of time than was necessary to produce overt malignancies. That would definitively prove the environmental nature of the disease, a cause and effect that no one could ignore.

The tobacco industry, the skeptics and unconvinced individuals, also those few physicians who, ignoring the science of their own profession, still were maintaining well into the sixties that the long time lag necessary for malignancies to develop, as well as the fact that apparently not everyone who smoked developed lung cancer, proved that smoking was not the cause of this disease, or at the very least not the sole cause, would finally have to agree with the committee's findings. If precancerous cells could be found in the lungs of smokers— even those who had only smoked for a few years—and not in the lungs of nonsmokers, then the proof would be there and the lack of overt malignancies in those who smoked would not be the rule but rather the exception.

The tobacco companies would then be in the position of having to explain why those people with already present premalignant lesions did not develop overt malignancies, why these didn't develop into cancer, not the other way around. The shoe would be on the other foot; the tobacco companies, instead of pointing to the seeming fact that not every smoker developed cancer, would have to explain why more didn't.

In 1958 it was found that 30 percent of boys, ranging from 18 percent in grade 9 to 40 percent in grade 12, and 17 percent of girls, ranging from 6 percent in grade 9 to 31 percent in

grade 12, had become cigarette smokers. The overall percentage was 14.7 for adolescent boys and 8.4 for adolescent girls.
The question was obvious: How dangerous was smoking to
these children? It was equally obvious that no one who remained unconvinced about the dangers of cigarette smoking
would accept another animal experiment; to make people listen, the precancerous changes had to be found in human lungs.

Two years later the proof of its danger was established in
the most drastic human experiments ever conceived, to prove
the carcinogenic effects of an environmental toxin. It was a
pathological study; young men dead before their time were
autopsied to try to save those not yet born or just beginning
to live. Since a diagnosis of lung cancer in adults was and still
is essentially a diagnosis of death, it seemed appropriate that
death itself should be used to prove a cause of dying.

O. Auerbach, the pathologist who devised the study, examined the lungs of 339 men who had been killed in industrial
accidents, slaughtered on the highways, murdered in holdups
or during arguments, dead from infections or cerebral hemor-
haging. These young men, pronounced dead from causes other
than pulmonary-induced disease, were autopsied, and at the
autopsy had their supposedly still healthy lungs removed and
examined. Detailed, extensive smoking histories were obtained
from relatives and friends. The data on time, duration,
amount, kinds of cigarettes smoked by these men were all
collected and tabulated.

Up to fifty-five blocks of lung tissue were removed from each
dead person, and number-coded. Each of the blocks was sectioned to a thickness of four microns, and the hundreds of
individual slides microscopically examined. Hundreds of sections were made from each block, each section thoroughly
stained and the stained tissues scrupulously studied.

What Auerbach and his associates looked for in these lung

sections were any signs of premalignant or malignant cellular change, no matter how early or how minute. What they found was the final unequivocal proof that cigarette smoking did indeed cause lung cancer, that all the data derived from hundreds of animal studies applied to man. Scattered throughout the tissues of these numbered blocks were found areas of precancerous transformations. It was a blind study; the pathologists involved had no idea whose lungs they were examining, or what the smoking history was of the men whose tissues they were looking at under the microscopes. They simply chronicled the cellular changes they saw.

When the microscopic part of the study was over, the codes finally broken and the results checked against the smoking histories of the men whose lungs had been removed and sectioned, the precancerous cellular changes that had been discovered were found almost entirely in the blocks of those who had smoked. The degree of malignant degeneration present was definitely related to the length of time and the number of cigarettes the person had smoked before his nonpulmonary death. Even after only a few years of smoking, premalignant cells were found lining the walls of the smokers' airways, strange-looking cells, their nuclei slightly distorted, their cytoplasm staining a bit more darkly, sitting there surrounded by still normal cells.

No standard errors here, no variances, no questionnaires to be filled out. The pathological study proved beyond dispute that inhaled tobacco smoke caused exposed cells to become premalignant, and that with more years of exposure or just irritation by an initiator substance—perhaps even the heat from the smoke itself, or the co-carcinogens in the particular matter of tobacco, or just the irritants in the air of urban areas —these cells suddenly become overtly malignant. Berenblum and Rous had proved thirty years ago that once cells become premalignant, they stay that way. With cancer it is only a question of time.

What applies to males, of course, holds equally for women. Writing on "Changing Epidemiology of Lung Cancer, Increasing Incidence in Women," in *Medical Clinics of North America* (1975), John Beamis states: "Significant numbers of women did not begin smoking cigarettes until the years before World War II; however, by 1960, nearly 40 percent of the women in the United States were smoking. From the experience in men, a rise could be predicted in the incidence of lung cancer in women twenty to thirty years after the large number of women began smoking. Our data bears this out, showing an increase in lung cancer death rates among women since 1960. The mortality curve for women is now similar to that of men in 1930."

As recently as September 1975, the *American Journal of Public Health* carried an article entitled "The Growing Epidemic. A survey of smoking habits and attitudes towards smoking among students grades 7 through 12." The article stated that "the increased smoking among boys and particularly girls in a recent 7 year period is of epidemic proportion. The striking and discouraging finding of our survey is the steep rise in smoking of children."

7.

And it is not only lung cancer. Nicotine by itself causes significant increases in heart rates and blood pressures as well as constriction of coronary arteries, all prerequisites for heart attacks. Smoking has also been linked to the development of bladder cancer. In their paper titled "Smoking and Cancer of the Lower Urinary Tract" (published in the *New England*

Journal of Medicine), authors Cole, Monsen and Hening stated: "It [smoking] appears to be the major factor associated with bladder cancer in the United States, considerably overshadowing any other factors."

Smoking by mothers has now been linked by Dr. Bergman of the Children's Orthopedic Hospital of Seattle to sudden death of their babies in infancy. Moreover, it is not only adults and infants who are affected by cigarette smoking, but the unborn as well. It is now universally agreed among neonatologists and public health officials, if not yet understood by the general public, that smoking during pregnancy interferes with fetal development.

If a mother smokes or is even constantly exposed to smoke-filled rooms, she will in all probability produce smaller babies, and have a one-third greater chance than a nonsmoking mother of giving birth to a stillborn. It is claimed by reputable scientists that the nicotine in the inhaled cigarette smoke is absorbed into the mother's circulation through her lungs, and crossing the placenta, interferes with the cells lining the blood supplies to the fetus, constricting those fetal blood vessels as it does the coronary arteries of adults, leading not to heart attacks but to a slowing down of the blood flow to the baby and in some instances, depending on the severity of the constriction, completely stopping it. A fetus needs an adequate blood supply to grow properly; any decrease in the supply for any reason will lead to congenital defects, delayed growth, retardation and even death.

It is not only a question of infant deaths, but children's health. Recently in England, three researchers—F.R.T. Colley, W.W. Holland and R.T. Corkhill—studying the incidence of pneumonia and bronchitis in 2,205 children during their first five years of life found that the incidence of pneumonia and bronchitis was highest in families where both parents smoked. They reported that exposure of infants to cigarette smoke doubled the risk of a pneumonia or bronchitis attacks.

Two other researchers, verifying Colley, Holland and Corkhill's report, showed that infants of smokers did indeed have significantly more admissions to hospitals than infants of non-smoking parents. Not only was there an increased number of hospitalizations for bronchitis and pneumonia in these exposed children, but also an increased admission rate for gastroenteritis, infections and inflammatory diseases. There is evidence that cigarette smoke absorbed through the lungs interferes with a person's immune system, decreasing the body's ability to fight off viral infections and kill invading bacteria. In the United States, O'Connell and Logan, studying childhood asthma at the Mayo Clinic, concluded that those parents who allowed their children exposure to cigarette smoke aggravated their children's condition.

The only conclusion that can be drawn from all this work, leaving aside the issue of adult cancers and heart attacks, is that embryos, infants and children exposed to cigarette smoke are being poisoned.

As a specialty, pediatrics owes its beginnings to a concern for adequate nutrition, appropriate housing and control of diarrheal diseases. It is a specialty that grew out of the realm of public health and preventive medicine. Its obligation, the task it has always taken upon itself, is the same now as always—to protect and to warn.

In the 1976 *Year Book of Pediatrics*, the editors, after evaluating most of the data on the effects of cigarette smoke on infants and children, sum up their concerns about the dangers of such exposure with the statement: "It seems wise to discourage parents from smoking if only for the sake of the health of their children."

The tobacco industry, the government, the Food and Drug Administration, the Department of Health, Education and Welfare, all have the same information the Surgeon General has—they have all read the Advisory Committee's reports, the articles on the dangers of smoking, the relationship of cigarettes to birth defects, stillborns, asthma, pneumonia, heart attacks, gastroenteritis, emphysema and bronchitis. They all know the studies on lung and bladder cancers. Smoking is today by far the major health problem in this country. Yet cigarette consumption is higher now than it was ten years ago. More women are smoking, more children and more adolescents are smoking now than ever before. Infants continue to be admitted to hospitals wheezing and coughing. Asthmatics sitting next to smokers or walking into smoke-filled rooms continue to suffer, and mothers continue to give birth to prematures and stillborns.

The obvious answer is to ban cigarettes in the same way that companies have been prohibited from selling bacterially contaminated foods or industries from dumping their poisonous wastes into our water supply. But profits, payoffs and investments continue to win out. The biases, prejudices and propaganda of the tobacco industry continue to succeed, the government continues to consent, and we continue to be ill and to die.

Since the right to smoke is allowed to take precedence over the right to health, it has to be every man and woman for himself and for his own. If the government in the name of personal freedom won't protect us, we must protect ourselves. The right to live, to health, is in everyone's own hands.

If your child has asthma, you have no choice but to insist that any smoker near him in a store, restaurant or wherever stop smoking. It is not the smoker, but you, who will have to take the time off from work to bring your child to the doctor, nor is it he who will have to pay for the possible hospitalization; you are the one who will have to stay up at night holding your child's hand while he tries to breathe, it is you, not he, who will have to go to the drugstore at two in the morning to get the cough medicine.

Nor does it end there. If you are a grandmother or a husband, you have no choice, if you want to be sure that you have a healthy baby born to your granddaughter or wife, but to insist that there be no smoking during the pregnancy, and that others who come in contact with the prospective mother stop smoking too. It has been shown that the amount of smoke inhaled by nonsmokers in a smoke-filled room is equivalent to their each smoking two or three cigarettes themselves. That is where it all stands now; if we care enough, we must simply begin to protect our own.

Yet there will always be those who, while perhaps willing to save others, are quite content to slowly kill themselves. Freedom has its price, though, and if a person wishes to smoke and to kill himself, if not others, he should at the very least be made to pay his own way. If someone smokes cigarettes long enough and deep enough, his lungs will eventually become malignant; he will begin to lose weight, cough up blood and be admitted to the hospital. Someone will have to pay for the admission, for the hospitalization, the operation, the chemotherapy, the follow-up care and the burial.

We know from the charts and tables approximately how many people will be hospitalized for lung cancer over the next three years. We know from the statistics so maligned by the tobacco industry that there will be at least 80,000 people stricken this year, 90,000 the next, and over 100,000 the year after that. We also know that of these hundreds of thousands, fewer than 5 percent will be alive one year after they are told they have cancer, and virtually none four years after that. We know, too, the number of procedures that will have to be performed on each patient, the average length of each hospital stay, the approximate daily cost of the hospitalization—at present a minimum of $150 a day anywhere in the country—and we know the cost in dollars and cents, if not tears and heartache, of all the follow-up care and medications.

For just one lung cancer patient, discounting the family's grief and loss of income, the emotional stresses in the surviving members and psychological burdens, the monetary cost is over $10,000; for the 80,000 of this year alone it will be $800 million. Next year it will be another billion. We know all this and each of us must share in these astronomical costs by having to pay in one way or another for those who refuse to listen to the warnings.

We know, too, from the tobacco industry's own figures how many packs of cigarettes are sold each year, and from the tobacco companies' figures we can project estimates of future sales—over 6.5 billion cigarettes next year alone. In the most modest of proposals, the people who insist on smoking should at least pay for their own deaths; others should not have to. The estimated medical bill for lung cancer over the next five years, not counting production losses as well as the medical personnel and resources that could be used elsewhere, will average $1 billion per year. These yearly anticipated costs could be divided by the yearly estimate of cigarettes to be sold, and that amount added to the sale price per pack. The Treasury Department could collect the added revenue and put it into a special cancer payment fund distributed through Medicare, if not through a special part of the newly proposed catastrophic-illness bill.

But we can't even wait for that. There is really no time. A recent editorial in the prestigious journal *Pediatrics* stated that pediatricians must take it upon themselves to deal with the dangers of smoking in the same way that they deal with the dangers of the infectious plagues. The editorial, the first of its kind, states that the health hazards of smoking must be discussed with each new set of parents at the same time and with the same force as the discussion of the need for immunization; that there is no difference between protecting a child from the ravages of measles, diphtheria or polio and protecting him from cigarette smoke.

VII

Hidden
Poisons

1.

You may never have heard of aflatoxin, but you could have been killed by it. Thousands already have been, and thousands more in India, Africa and the Philippines are dying because of it right now even as you read this page.

Aflatoxin is a chemical substance produced by *Aspergillus flavus,* a mold similar to the one that produces the antibiotic penicillin. But unlike penicillin, the chemical produced by aspergillus does not inhibit bacterial growth. It causes cancer.

Aspergillus flavus under warm moist conditions will grow on any vegetable food. The mold itself is a natural contaminant of nuts or practically any processed meal, but especially improperly processed peanuts. It was first discovered as a carcinogen in England, where literally overnight almost every turkey in the country died from being fed grain contaminated by the mold. The deaths alerted health officials to the poisonous, though at that time still unknown, dangerous nature of the grain. At autopsy the only abnormality found was restricted solely to the birds' livers. Their livers were found to be completely destroyed, their liver cells totally ruined. Great concern developed over the possibility of human consumption of similar grains, and work was begun immediately to determine exactly what had killed the birds.

It was soon found that the grain was not the cause, but rather the aspergillus growing on the grain, and ultimately that it was not even the contaminating mold but the aflatoxin it produced which had caused the turkey's deaths by poisoning their livers. The veterinarians found the feed so overgrown with mold that it had become saturated with the chemical; once the turkeys began to eat the grain they ingested so much of the toxin that their liver cells became acutely poisoned and the birds died not of cancer but of liver failure. The heavily contaminated feed was removed from the market, and the problem considered solved. It wasn't.

At the same time, trout being raised in hatcheries in the United States were suddenly found to be developing liver cancers. It was discovered that they too had been fed grain contaminated with the aspergillus mold, but that their feed, not so heavily contaminated by the mold as that fed to the turkeys, had not killed them. Instead the trout, eating small amounts, even minute amounts of the toxin, developed cancers in their livers, dying slowly from liver malignancies rather than quickly, as the birds had, from acute liver failure.

What the trout and turkey breeders learned was what cancer researchers had known for some time: carcinogens are cellular poisons. Taken in large amounts they so widely disrupt or destroy intracellular machinery that they cause cellular death; in small amounts they let cells live, but interfering or coupling with subcellular control mechanisms, cause cancer.

In areas of Africa below the Sahara and in India, small amounts of aspergillus have continually been found in grains eaten by humans; metabolites of aflatoxin have been identified in the urine of children eating these contaminated products.

What happened to the trout has happened to people. The highest incidence of liver cancer in the world is found in those populations eating aspergillus-contaminated food. Study after study in Swaziland and Papua, among the Kikuyus in East Africa and in Bangladesh show an increased incidence of death from liver cancer in humans eating as little as one billionth of a gram of aflatoxin a day. These people died from amounts of toxin so minute, so tiny as to be undetectable with anything less than the most sophisticated medical sensors.

If no one you know has ever died from liver cancer due to the ingestion of aflatoxin, it is not because of billions spent on cancer research, or the establishment of liver-cancer-detection centers, or even the development of better liver-cancer therapy. Why? It is because our meal products are tested and the sale of contaminated grains prohibited. None of our cancer surgeons talk today of an epidemic of liver cancers in this country, celebrities don't pose with children wasting away from hepatic tumors, there are no liver-cancer wards because we have stopped the disease by simply not letting it occur.

Others have not been so lucky. People in Africa, India and the Philippines continue to die from malignancies of the liver. They continue to eat the microscopically contaminated grains, and like the trout, slowly perish, dying from what they are fed. Sooner or later liver cells continually exposed to this low-grade carcinogen turn malignant, and then the bone pain follows, the bloody vomiting and the diarrhea, the wasting away and finally death.

2.

If you were a scientist engaged in cancer research and wanted —indeed, had no choice because of limited research funds— to be sure that every rat used in your experiments developed cancer, you would simply feed them nitrosamines. You could purchase the chemical from any one of the number of biological supply houses or commercial laboratories scattered around the country. Or, if you wanted to save even more money, you could make your own by simply taking a few grams of inexpensive nitrites, mixing them in a test tube with some easily obtained amines, and heating the combination over a Bunsen burner.

Whenever nitrites come in contact with amines, they combine to form a new stable chemical compound called nitrosamine. You can use different kinds of amines and get different kinds of nitrosamines—and depending on the nitrosamine, you can produce different kinds of cancers in rats. You can even heat up nitrites with special amines to form nitrosamines that will cross the placenta of pregnant animals and cause cancer in their fetuses.

All of this would be of little general interest if it were not for the fact that what the researcher can do in his laboratory to produce nitrosamines occurs every day in the processed meats you eat.

The latest estimates available indicate that nitrites (or nitrates—both compounds being essentially the same, since nitrites are oxidized in the presence of air to nitrates) are added to billions of pounds of this country's meat products each year.

All meats contain amines; they result from the normal decay of meat proteins. The number of these amines constantly increases as the meats gradually age. When this happens, the nitrites added by the processor to your bologna and salami, bacon and liver loaf slowly combine with the ever increasing amounts of amines, producing nitrosamines. Nothing can stop the reaction. Just as in the researcher's test tube, once the nitrites come into contact with the amines, the nitrosamines are formed. All the scientist did in his laboratory by adding heat to the test tube containing the amines and nitrites was speed up the process of conversion. You may cook your processed meat, fry the salami, heat the bacon, make a corned-beef omelette, but what you are getting is what the researcher gets when he heats his test tubes—more nitrosamines.

Recently the U.S. Department of Agriculture found traces of nitrosamines in three of forty-eight samples of processed meat studied. In tests conducted by the FDA, nitrosamines were found in one out of sixty hams tested. A known carcinogen, measureable, was already there in some of the processed meats we are all eating.

The authoritative *Medical Drug Letter,* a publication devoted to the uncompromising evaluation of new drugs, put the issue of nitrosamines—which it considers for all practical purposes a drug—into an unusually clear if decidedly academic perspective:

"Conversion of nitrates to nitrite is enhanced when nitrate-containing foods spoil, but it also occurs slowly in any food that is not vacuum packed. Nitrates are added to more than 12 billion pounds of food every year in the U.S. The highest concentrations are found in hot dogs, bacon, ham, lunch meats, smoked fish and imported cheeses. In the United States the Food and Drug Administration limits residual nitrites to 200 parts per million. When foods are spotchecked, however, considerably more nitrites have been found repeatedly. Large amounts of nitrites are considered potentially dangerous because nitrites combine with amines in human stomachs or alone to form nitrosamines. Nitrosamines are also formed from secondary amines and quarternary ammonium compounds found in food and drugs. . . . Nitrosamines themselves have been found in food, especially bacon after frying. . . . Tumors have been induced in a wide range of animals by most of these substances. Nitrosamines may also be mutagenic causing muta-

tions and teratogenic causing congenital malformations. . . .
Eating foods containing nitrites may lead to the formation of
nitrosamines, which are carcinogen in animals and could well
act similarly in man."

Millions, perhaps even billions of dollars are spent each year
in medical and surgical departments throughout the country in
doing research on animals under the accepted and proven
theory that what occurs in animals is medically and surgically
applicable to people. Diseases are produced in rats, mice and
guinea pigs, and then new drugs, hopefully destined for human
use, are given to determine if the experimentally induced diseases can be halted or cured, while operative procedures devised to treat human conditions are first tested on dogs, cats,
baboons and chimpanzees. Federal, state and private monies
support this kind of research with the understanding that if the
drugs or procedures work in animals, they will be useful in
humans.

Virtually all our understanding of the processes involved in
human disease and treatment has come from animal studies.
We cannot have it both ways. We cannot accept a closeness
with animals in only those things we wish to have, and ignore
the closeness in those things that make us uncomfortable. We
cannot accept for our children the newest congenital-heart
operations developed in dogs, or the newest high-blood-pres-
sure medication proven in rabbits, and then try to convince
ourselves that after all, we really are different from these animals. We aren't. The Dicumarol that poisoned our babies
poisoned rats; the thalidomide that kept babies' arms and legs
from growing crippled baby chimps as well. Down at the cellular level we are all really the same; there is absolutely no reason
to assume that what causes animals' cells to turn malignant will
not cause our cells to do the same, that the nitrosamines which
produce cancers in rats will not produce the cancers in us.

Berenblum's experiments proved that a carcinogen can cause malignant transformation in much lower concentration than expected if in one way or another a promoting substance is also involved. The implications for the carcinogens we now know we are exposed to are plain. With the nitrosamines in our diet, the promoters might well be the spices, the salt and pepper, in our food, or even the gastric irritation that follows an alcoholic binge, perhaps even the irritation of aspirin ingestion.

Tobacco companies have argued for years that the concentration of the carcinogen in the coal tars of tobacco smoke was too low to be of any real concern. Now they push low-tar cigarettes, when the truth is that Berenblum's discoveries, confirmed by others, showed that practically any exposure to a carcinogen is dangerous because of promoter effects.

The same argument about concentrations of carcinogens has been used by the food industry in regard to its preservatives and food colorings. This argument forms the background for all the industry-backed comments about people having to eat carloads of cancer-producing substances before they could possibly develop cancers. Indeed, it has become the argument used by practically every industry that has been pumping carcinogens directly into each of us or into the environment in general.

But over fifty years of continuing experimentation has proved and proved again that the amount of carcinogen necessary to produce cancers can be minute and still be deadly. Industry likes to push the idea of a threshold to carcinogenic exposures—a lower limit of exposure that is not dangerous. This concept of a threshold forms the basis for industry's repudiation of animal studies where animals are fed what they say are huge amounts of materials, the "boxcar" equivalents that they say humans could never consume. Recently, though, Dr. James Watson, the Nobel Prize-winner, answered that concern by stating that in truth there may be no threshold to carcinogenic exposures—that it is scientifically possible that one molecule of a carcinogen getting into a cell and penetrating the nucleus could damage any DNA molecule enough to change it, to cause the cell to lose control and become malignant. Industry has never been able to prove otherwise. If companies were honest or concerned, they would either have to be silent about the potential harmfulness of their products or admit that all the scientific evidence available proves that even minute exposures to known cancer-causing agents, with or without promoters, can be harmful, and that there is not one single bit of experimental or clinical evidence indicating anything else.

3.

In 1956 an international conference of scientists in Rome declared Red Dye #2 to be a suspected carcinogen. Under increasing challenge in the United States as a cancer-causing agent, this same dye was only recently cleared by the Food and Drug Administration for unlimited use in foodstuffs. But so much pressure was brought to bear, so much opposition generated by consumer groups that the agency subsequently reversed itself and late in 1975 banned further use of the chemical in new products, but allowed the continued sale of any products that contained the dye before the ban. It is still there in the food we are eating.

The dye's real name is amaranth, and for all that the food industry may have said in its defense, it is a derivative of coal tars. It had been added to billions of dollars' worth of food annually for no other reason than that it hides blemishes and makes low-quality food look more expensive, more appetizing. It was even added to dog food to make that product more appealing—not to dogs but to buyers, since it has been known for years that all dogs are color-blind. The dye's sole purpose was to deceive or to entice, and for those two purposes we were poisoning ourselves—or to be more exact, we were being poisoned.

While Red Dye # 2 was being added to our foods, the Soviet Union banned its use in their own. West Germany's authorities limited its use in their country to certain foods, and the World Health Organization recommended world-wide limitations so strict that if implemented, they would essentially eliminate the use of the dye in all foodstuffs.

The Russians based the banning of Red Dye # 2 on their 1971 study which concluded that the dye caused cancer in laboratory animals. The FDA itself, in a study done a few years later but never published, in which rats had Red Dye # 2 added to their feed, confirmed the Russian view. The report stated: "The only effect of any consequence attributable to the colors [three other dyes were studied separately] was the increase, roughly a doubling, in the number of breast tumors with three of the four colors." One of the three was Red Dye # 2.

An FDA statistician, after reviewing the data from the FDA study, wrote: "The study offers grounds for suspicion that there is a cancerous effect of the dye." Other scientists agreed. Dr. H. L. Stewart of the National Cancer Institute commented: "There was a suspicion that the colors [among them Red Dye # 2] were increasing the incidence of breast tumors [in animals fed the dye]." An internal FDA memo concerning the agency's own studies stated: "Statistically, the [Red Dye # 2] mice had significantly more total tumors than did the controls." The Russian study put it even more simply: "Chemically pure amaranth possesses carcinogenic activity of medium strength and should not be used in food industry."

The amount of food in the United States to which Red Dye

2 was added exceeded in sales the total yearly profits from the whole prescription-drug market. As a nation we consumed more amaranth in twelve months than we did the antibiotics ampicillin and tetracycline put together. Over one and a half million pounds of pure amaranth a year was used. Made from coal tars, materials known to be carcinogenic ever since the first observation of cancers developing in the skins of chimney sweeps, the dye was added to just about everything consumable, ranging from lipstick to pill coatings. It was used in non-cola drinks, candy bars, gelatin desserts and baked goods, syrups, cake and pudding mixes, breakfast cereals, cold meats, hot dogs, sausages, vinegar, salad dressings, pretzels, corn chips, sweet rolls, ice cream, processed meats, cakes and jams. Because it produced a durable, almost perfect red, it was used even in liquid medicines, not to make them taste better, but to make them look better.

A recent vice president for corporate research at General Foods summed up in a memo the food industry's one concern about the chemical: "We're down to three usable red colors now and if they ban Red No. 2 we're dangerously close to having no reds at all. Without it grape drinks look muddy. People don't want to buy food that does not look like it always looked."

An industry observer explained the position of the producers in dealing with the Congress and with health agencies: "The strategy was to force delay after delay on a determination, in this case restrictions on the dye, in the hopes that it finally fizzles out." Yet while the industry, obviously feeling no responsibility for anything other than profit, was hoping people would forget, more data on the dangers of the dye were being accumulated.

Since most carcinogens are by their nature mutagens—that is, they do their damage to cells by injuring the cells' genetic material—then theoretically Red Dye # 2, a carcinogen, should also cause birth defects if given to embryos. It soon became evident that it did. The FDA might have ignored its own test indicating the carcinogenicity of the dye as well as the Russian tests supporting that view, but they were truly alarmed when additional Soviet tests linked the dye to fetal toxicity. After all, cancers take twenty years and more to develop, but any mother who sees her child being born deformed, without arms and legs, without eyes or with a twisted spine, is going to demand an accounting. Even industry pressures fade away in front of a constituency of furious parents holding their malformed children in their arms.

Red Dye # 2 was discovered to cause fetal toxicity when Shutenberg and Bavrilenko, two Russians testing the drug, found that it caused fetal deaths if administered to pregnant rats in doses of as little as 1.5 milligrams per kilogram of body weight per day. Collins in the United States found statistically significant fetal toxicity at levels of 30 mg/kg. Tests on another animal, the rabbit, showed again that Red Dye # 2 in dosages as low as 1.5 mg/kg resulted in increased fetal resorption.

The first experiment conducted by the FDA on the fetal toxicity of Red Dye # 2 was begun in the spring of 1971. Chick embryos were injected with small quantities of the dye. The results are still available today preserved in jars of formalin; baby chicks with oversized eyes and twisted skeletons, absent limbs and grotesquely shaped heads. But like blind men, the FDA refused to accept the results as conclusive. They complained that their own experiments did not fit into standard dose response relationships, that the study was too small and the amount of dye used too great. The results were simply not accepted as conclusive by the agency.

In a terrible ignoring of the public trust, the Food Protection Consultants of the federal government, faced with what any reasonable scientist would have considered ample evidence to ban Red Dye #2 at least until more definitive testing could be done, or at least to stop its continued addition to our food until more data could be obtained, simply allowed the company that manufactured the dye to continue to sell it, and food processers to add it to our food. Unable to explain away the Russian studies, or even their own statistics, the FDA, like the tobacco companies, denounced the testing methods used as inadequate, and ignored the cancers and the injured fetuses.

While lobbyists bombarded agency officials and congressmen—"Do you know this [the banning of Red Dye #2] could ruin us economically?" "Would you like some eminent doctors to call you and testify that this dye is safe?"—it was being calculated that a 110-pound woman would absorb enough of this coal-tar derivative to reach dangerous blood levels by drinking as little as a third of a can of grape soda daily. A child could exceed the recognized safe limit with just a couple of gulps from the same can of pop. Collins and McLaughlin in their paper entitled "Teratology Studies of Food Colors: Embryo-Toxicity of Amaranth" stated that "Dose related feto-toxic response was obtained with Red Dye 2 which was statistically significant at and above the 30 mgm/kgm dose level."

Even if you as an individual had been concerned about Red Dye #2, and wanted to stop eating or drinking it yourself or stop having your family exposed to it, you couldn't because you had no way of knowing if you were ingesting it. Although the Federal Food, Drug and Cosmetic Act requires food manufacturers to state on their labels if artificial coloring is used, the type of dye does not have to be specified. Butter, cheese and ice cream are totally exempt from even this minor labeling requirement, these products not being required to list any coloring additives.

On the basis of the Russians' study alone on the toxicity of

Red Dye # 2 to fetuses, as well as the FDA's own "equivocal" results on fetal poisonings, the use of amaranth should have been banned years ago. In addition to these fetal studies, the carcinogenic concerns and the almost universal agreement among cancer researchers that no dose of a carcinogen can be determined as a safe dose, the chemical should have been summarily destroyed. Like aflatoxin-contaminated grains, food that contains Red Dye # 2 should have been dumped.

Yet even with the FDA's ban in force, foodstuffs containing Red Dye # 2 already on the shelves are allowed continued sale. Apparently profits come first, health second. At the very minimum, the public should know which of the food and beverages still allowed to be sold contain the dye so people can choose for themselves if they want to be exposed to a coal-tar derivative, for no other reason than to have a brighter maraschino cherry in their drinks, or a redder helping of strawberry ice cream.

Industry is now gearing up to use Red Dye # 40 in foods instead of Red Dye # 2. The issue is still the same and in truth Red Dye # 40 has already been banned in other countries of the world. Foolishness and greed go on; but perhaps after each new victory the battle against them gets easier, if not the war.

4.

No child we know of has as yet been born with the grotesque defects of the fetal chickens exposed to Red Dye # 2, nor has any group of children recently been born without the arms and legs of the thalidomide babies. But there are types of congenital defects more subtle, though equally as disastrous, as being born into this world overtly deformed. There are biological defects: children who should have been normal but are now slow learners, those with poor motor coordination, those who can't hear high-pitched sounds properly or can't speak correctly; those who invert their letters or can't read—all those children with the so-called "soft signs" of neurological impairment, which can be as great a cause of family heartache and grief as a child born with a congenital heart defect or malformed kidneys.

At a recent Senate committee hearing Dr. Benjamin Feingold, Chief Emeritus of the Allergy Department of the Kaiser-Permanente Medical Center in San Francisco, began to explain to the assembled senators the results of twenty-five years of his own work. His topic was hyperactive children and the connection between food additives and hyperactivity which he had discovered and had been pursuing virtually alone and unsupported for almost a quarter century. He started by reading a verbatim report:

" 'We were told he was allergic. We were told he was a screwball . . . but now when he wakes up in the morning his hair isn't all scruffed up in the back from tossing and turning. He doesn't grind his teeth. When you ask him a question you get a paragraph instead of an I don't wanna. He is able to concentrate.' "

What Feingold was quoting to the committee was the comments of a mother whose eleven-year-old son was neither allergic nor a screwball, but one of the five million children diagnosed in this country as being hyperactive.

The child's transformation was not the result of expensive psychiatric treatments, nor due to the drugs Ritalin or Benzedrine, but the result of being put on a diet free of artificial colors and artificial flavorings.

Feingold had discovered years before that in putting hyperactive children on diets that eliminated step by step most food additives, some of his patients gradually got better. The issue was again poison. A new textbook on pharmacology, soon to be published by the University of Minnesota, devotes a full chapter to the effects of additives on the brain, but back when Feingold began his work there was no such text to point to, no interest in the environmental nature of hyperactivity. People were looking for viruses, then childhood infections, minor trauma to the brain, and congenital defects as the cause for hyperactivity. His work was attacked as unscientific, uncontrolled, unstatistical and anecdotal.

Working by himself, trying to prove a new concept, Feingold had no defense against these attacks except to say that when you do not even know what you are dealing with, when the food additives children are exposed to number in the dozens, when companies wouldn't even tell you what is in their products—when ingredients listed under the general terms "enzymes" or "artificial coloring" and "preservatives" can mean virtually anything—the only scientific studies that can be employed are elimination studies. But the parents of those hyperactive children, faced with an observable immediate problem—an uncontrollable child and needing help—supported Feingold's work, as did the few doctors who realized that the drugs used for the treatment of this condition had side effects of their own.

Finally, after twenty years, the National Institute of Education, not the FDA, financed a study conducted by Dr. C. Keith Connors of the University of Pittsburgh which supported Feingold's theory about the effects of artificial colorings on brain cells. "Fifteen children were divided into two groups. One group received a control diet, which contained additives, and the other received an additive-free diet. Then each group changed diets. The children were not told what they were eating, but parents and teachers noticed a significant reduction of hyperactive symptoms when the children were on an additive-free diet."

No matter what arguments were used against Connors'

study—that there might have been nutritional deficiencies between the diets, lower carbohydrates in one than in the other —the important fact was that the diet changed these children's behavior for the better, that a new nonmedical method of treatment and prevention of a tragic childhood condition was available. The study indicated that at the very minimum, the idea of environmental toxins as a cause of hyperactivity should not be discarded, that more money and effort should be put into further research and study on the dietary control of this condition. "It is interesting to note," Feingold told the Senate committee, "that a graph projected for the estimated incidence of hyperkinesis [hyperactivity] and learning disabilities over the past ten years parallels the Standard & Poor curves for the dollar value for soft drinks and synthetic flavors over the same period."

It would seem as if drugs and food additivies are unrelated. They are not. In the nineteen-sixties, cobalt sulfate was added to certain beers when it was found that small amounts of this "additive" would cause the beer when poured to produce a bigger head. Within weeks several people drinking the beer were dead. Later it was found what had not been suspected or even tested for: that small amounts of cobalt when mixed with alcohol and ingested were toxic. Except for terminology, there is no difference between a compound taken as a drug and one ingested as an additive.

Dicumarol gets into liver cells, radioactive iodine into thyroids. There is no reason to assume that chemicals ingested as additives do not act in exactly the same way. The body does not differentiate between ingested substances, no matter what their labels. If a tranquilizer can get into brain cells and by disrupting their subcellular structures lead to erratic behavior, why should not food colorings do the same? Where there is any scientific indication that this can happen, studies to prove or disprove the fact must be pursued as diligently and as thoroughly as the studies into the causes of the infectious diseases were once pursued.

VIII

Cellular Toxins

1.

Epidemiology, the study of the causes of disease, is always an after-the-fact science. It deals with past disasters; its concern for the future arises from recognition of what has already happened. The discovery of German measles as the cause of birth defects had to await World War II with the clustering of women workers in factories before enough blind and deaf children were born in one area for the infectious origin of the defects to become obvious. We had to wait for similar disasters in the cases of drugs and pregnant women to point the way to the causes of congenital defects and the dangers of medicating pregnant women.

It is the same with cancers. Clusterings of malignancies in certain areas, an increased incidence of unusual cancers, cancers occurring where they shouldn't, in special groups of people, in people where they hadn't been found before, or even simply an increased incidence in the rate of routine, well-known types of malignancies—all these ring the alarm bell.

It was the sudden appearance of a rare type of cancer that

alerted health officials to the dangers of PVC, polyvinyl chloride. Like aflatoxin, PVC injures the liver. However, unlike aflatoxin, it is not ingested and absorbed into the bloodstream through the stomach, but through the skin or mucous membranes. Nor does it, like aflatoxin, injure the liver cells themselves, but the cells of the small blood vessels that line the liver. Polyvinyl chloride causes those small vessel cells to turn malignant, producing a particularly deadly form of cancer called angiosarcoma.

Why it is that those few small vessel cells of the liver and no others are affected by PVC no one knows. It must be for much the same reason that only certain fetal cells are affected by thalidomide, while still others are affected by Dilantin; something unique, some intracellular structure, some special hormone or enzyme in the cells lining the small vessels of the liver which are not in any of the other cells of the body, structures that the molecules of polyvinyl chloride or a metabolite of the chemical are able to couple with or injure so that years, even decades later, perhaps under the influence of some promoter, the cells suddenly change and turn overtly malignant.

There may well be no lower limits to the exposure to PVC that can cause angiosarcomas to develop. Until recently it was used as a propellant in hair sprays. Whether those short bursts of exposure in bathrooms or in front of hallway mirrors has already put at risk thousands of young women we can't yet be sure. But we know now that it was not only the men working in PVC factories and dying from angiosarcomas who paid the price for their exposures. It was also their wives and their children.

In a joint study of the National Institute for Occupational Safety and Health, the United States Center for Disease Control's Bureau of Epidemiology and the University of North

Carolina School of Public Health it was discovered that the wives of men who worked with PVC had twice the number of miscarriages or stillborns as wives of those whose husbands were not exposed.

The scientists of these bureaus studied the fetal death rates for women whose husbands worked at PVC-monomer plants, which produced the basic vinyl chemical, compared to the rates among women whose husbands worked in the rubber and PVC factories which turned the already solid plastic into consumer goods.

Before the husbands were exposed to the basic PVC-monomer, their wives had a fetal death rate of 6.1 per 100 pregnancies—below the rate experienced by women whose husbands worked in the relatively safer rubber and PVC plants. But after their husbands were exposed to the monomer gas, the fetal death rate shot up to 15.8 per 100.

Again, this discovery of fetal deaths came as no surprise to cancer researchers. For all the seeming difference between malignant transformation and congenital defects, between lung cancer and stillborns, the processes causing them are the same—cellular injury. When mature adult cells are exposed to nonlethal doses of a carcinogen, they turn malignant. When fetal cells having to form themselves into thousands of different kinds of tissues are similarly poisoned, replication errors are produced that lead to congenital defects, and in some cases childhood cancers as well.

A chemical that causes malignant transformations in mature cells can also poison exposed sex cells. The medical theory proposed for the increase in stillborns and miscarriages among children of the PVC workers is that the chemical entering the bodies of these men circulated not only to their livers but to their testes, where it damaged the developing sperm cells, producing such severe genetic injury to these cells' DNA that the child conceived by these "damaged" cells was doomed from its very beginnings. Unlike rabbits, which absorb their dead fetuses, humans give birth to them.

Yet polyvinyl chloride is still released into the air around the factories that produce it, and food wrapped in plastics made from PVC may well absorb small amounts of the chemical from the wrappings. We can eliminate the risk of angiosarcoma, as well as the risk of stillborns from PVC exposure, the same way we have lowered the risk of liver-cell cancers from exposure to aflatoxin by simply not allowing it.

2.

In the late fifties it was discovered that workers involved in the production of asbestos-cement fireproofing materials and insulation had rates of cancer ten times that of workers in other industries. Inhaled and ingested asbestos particles were found to be carcinogenic, causing lung cancer as well as a rare type of malignancy—mesotheliomas of the chest wall. The discovery of the carcinogenic nature of asbestos fibers, like the discovery of the malignant properties of polyvinyl chloride, was too late for the workers already dead; it was even too late for those who were not dead at the time of the discovery but had already been sufficiently exposed to be in risk of dying. But if proper protection is used, it is not too late for the children and adolescents who will someday work in those factories or even those adults who are starting today.

This has already happened in the shale and mineral-oil-exposed industries. Workers whose hands were turning malignant led doctors to realize the carcinogenic nature of these industrial oils. These cancers were eliminated by having the workers wear protective clothing and gloves. Health officials demanded the clothing, and now no workers' hands turn malignant.

By simple elementary prevention, one cancer after another has been eliminated, wiped from the earth as surely and completely as smallpox and cholera.

In the early nineteen-forties it was discovered that workers in aniline-dye factories had an abnormally high incidence of bladder cancers. In many instances these lethal tumors had apparently not developed until twenty years after exposure, and in some cases even longer. The same extended period between exposure and tumor production has been found in almost all the other environmentally induced human cancers, as it had been observed in practically all experimental animal studies. Angiosarcomas from PVC exposure, mesotheliomas from asbestos, liver cancers from aflatoxin—all took fifteen to twenty-five years after initial exposure to develop.

Again as with Berenblum's animal studies, the original exposure did not have to be of long duration. Some men who developed malignancies of their bladders due to aniline dyes had worked in those dye factories for as little as two or three years, and then went on to other jobs that never again brought them into contact with any other carcinogenics. Obviously the cells of these men's bladders had undergone a premalignant transformation during their brief exposure in the factory, only to turn overtly cancerous years later, perhaps under the influence of some promoter that found its way into the urine that bathed these worker's bladders.

Because of protective measures, there is no longer any general exposure to aniline dyes. Yet bladder cancers account today for 4 percent of all the malignancies in the United States, totaling 40,000 to 60,000 new cases a year. Reason, if not common sense, demands that where the cause for a disease has been found, and where that disease still persists or increases, similar causes should be looked for. If exposure to aniline dyes have proved to cause bladder cancers, why shouldn't exposure to other industrial chemicals do the same thing? Apparently they do. The highest incidence of bladder cancer in this country is in the industrialized Northeast, and the highest incidence of all is in New Jersey, the nation's most industrialized state. We know already that as little as .0000000000002 ounces of aflatoxin ingested per day leads to liver cancer. The waters in New Jersey are foul with chemical wastes. If human exposures to aniline dyes that entered the bloodstream and concentrated in the bladder of aniline-dye workers caused cancer, why not the bathing of other bladder cells in other industrial products? Yet there are researchers who continually ask Congress for millions of dollars so that they can find the virus that supposedly causes bladder cancers, while they ignore what to any reasonable scientists would be the most logical target of investigations—chemical pollutants.

One of the country's best-known urologists, a man who operates every week on people with bladder cancers, recently confided, "Sure, of course, they may all be caused by carcinogens. You'd think the people most involved would be the most helpful, most concerned about finding out if they are, but we get no cooperation at all from industry. The rubber companies, whose workers are constantly exposed to solvents and dyes, adhesives and irritants, wouldn't even release their data on the incidence of bladder cancers among their own workers. They wouldn't cooperate in any of our proposed studies; none of them will. The workers won't be dead until later, anyway, after they've done their work."

Arsenicals once distributed widely as tonics but found to cause skin cancers are not allowed to be sold any more. But the workers in copper smelters where arsenic is produced as a by-product of copper production are still exposed. In the late nineteen-sixties a report published by a copper-industry physician, a doctor employed and paid for by the smelter company, indicated no increased incidence of cancer among the plant's exposed workers. The report, which was accepted by federal, state and local regulatory agencies as fact, was later proved to be totally erroneous, at worst a fabrication, at best a complete distortion of the standardized medical coding procedures used by medical statisticians and hospital registrars all over the world. When the death certificates of the smelter workers were rechecked by public health officials, it was found that the incidence of lung cancer among those workers had been increasing for years. The culpability of the smelter officials and the physicians employed by the company will be left to history or the courts; the real issue is that the men working in those plants continue to be exposed to the arsenic dust, continue to develop lung cancers, and continue to die.

The plant is still running; workers are still being exposed, and a whole new generation of young workers will soon have malignant changes occurring in their lungs. There is no need for any research here, for extensive biological laboratories, or additional surveys to find out why these men are dying. No experimental animals are needed to confuse the issue; the ultimate experiment has already been done. Men have died; the rest can be saved by merely stopping their exposure and another cancer will be gone.

3.

There is, unfortunately, a natural course to any new discovery. There is always that first initial burst of enthusiasm and euphoria, the backslapping, the pride and the arrogance, the great plans and widespread usage; then, slowly, the complications begin, the errors that initially weren't thought of, the dangers that hadn't been anticipated. They occur at first as isolated events, seemingly random, one complication here, another there. But as the new discovery is more widely accepted or more commonly employed, the complications become more frequent and more severe until finally dissatisfaction and disillusionment set in.

The new discovery is then either totally disregarded, as were some of the operative techniques of the early sixties, or a new and more realistic balance is reached in which the benefits of the discovery are weighed against its risks. Chloromycetin kills microbes but was also found to cause allergies and severe bone-marrow depressions, sometimes even death, so its use is now restricted to special severe microbial infections. Television gives wide coverage to events but leaves little time for evaluation and thought, so people have learned to question its interpretations. Cars move us better than horses, but we have learned we must protect ourselves from their pollution.

That's the way it was with radium. The discovery that there were rocks which luminesce in the dark and emitted rays that pass through solid objects, leaving the objects' shape imprinted on photographic film, was met initially with wonder and enthusiasm. The rocks were purified and the radioactive material obtained given the name of radium. The wonder remained but the enthusiasm soon began to wane.

The fact that purified radium would brightly luminesce in the dark was quickly picked up by the watch industry as a means of nighttime illumination for their watch faces. In the thirties, workers were employed to sit at benches with little bottles of radium-based paint in front of them as they painted the numerals on the watch dials. They soon learned what artists had known for centuries, that to paint tiny objects the tip of the brush must be kept firm and fine, and the only way to do that without continually interrupting work is to moisten the brush point with the lips.

The radium worker would dip his brush in the radium, paint the numeral, lick the brush to get back its point, and then dip the brush again in the radium bottle, paint another numeral, put the brush back in the mouth to set its point and then begin again. During each of these cycles a minute amount of radium would be licked off the brush, and entering the painter's mouth, be absorbed through his mucous membranes into the bloodstream. Years later their bones would begin to degenerate and the workers would die of bone cancer and leukemias.

The same series of events, the same initial enthusiasm followed by the same unexpected disasters occurred with fluoroscopy. The original X-ray machines were soon adapted not only to take static films of patients' insides but to follow organ functions as well. With the use of X-ray–dense materials like barium the new machines could scan for minutes on end, following gastric motility, looking for ulcers in the upper GI tract and polyps in the rectum. But the patients had to be moved around to make the fluoroscope effective, different views continually had to be taken to ensure all parts of the organs under examination were seen. The first radiologists with total enthusiasm and confidence in their new machines moved their patients around themselves. They even held them while the machines were working, with their own uncovered hands continually exposed to the high-energy beams. There was patient after patient, examination after examination.

After a time little sores began to appear on the physicians' fingers and hands. The sores were at first dismissed as unimportant, but they wouldn't heal and gradually they got worse. Eventually the sores began to ulcerate, exposing muscles and tendons, and then the fingers themselves began slowly to erode and eventually the tips had to be surgically removed. But again the same sores appeared at the margins of the surgical amputations. Operation followed operation, mutilation followed mutilation. The sores were discovered to be skin cancers, caused by the radiologists' having exposed their hands to the high-energy beams of their own machines. Eventually many were to die with nothing left of their upper limbs but oozing stumps.

Workers don't die any more from radium poisoning. Their bones no longer turn malignant, nor do the hands of workers exposed to industrial oils. Gloves and lead aprons put an end to radiologists' becoming amputees, just as the stopping of the irradiation of chest and neck of infants has put an end to what is now a common type of thyroid cancer. Three different malignancies—bone cancer, thyroid malignancies and squamous-cell carcinomas of the skin—have all been conquered without billions of dollars being spent, stopped by the elimination of carcinogenic exposures by nothing more than adequate protection, by simply not allowing ourselves to be poisoned.

IX

The Ames Test

1.

We have learned the ways to stop disease, and it can be stopped; it is not at all a hopeless task. Surgeons do it every day when they sterilize their surgical instruments, hospital aides do it when they scrub down operating-room walls and use disinfectants to clean out respirators and dialysis machines.

Disease can be stopped in any number of ways. It can be stopped by destroying its carriers. Walter Reed accomplished this seventy years ago by destroying the mosquitoes that transmitted yellow fever, and today we still do it by destroying the mosquitoes that carry malaria. If the infecting organism is too mobile to be caught, too powerful, or has no carrier, we can gear up the body to make its own fight. No one ever kept one single polio virus from going where it pleased, nor has anyone ever with his own eyes even seen a live rabies microbe, yet through the use of vaccines these diseases are no longer a threat. Measles, mumps, typhoid, typhus, cholera, German measles have all been conquered in this way.

Against those diseases for which vaccines are not available

or haven't as yet been discovered we have developed pre-formed antibodies to give the body the time it needs to win. Tetanus injections of antitoxin supply the body with already made antibodies that attach to and couple with the infecting toxin, buying the body the time it needs to make its own antibodies, to win its own battle. Diphtheria antitoxin gives the body the same edge. Penicillin, streptomycin, polymyxin, Chloromycetin go after the microbes themselves, giving us the chance we need.

Yet no matter how dramatic it may seem, no disease treatment is 100 percent certain. No matter how high the temperature at which surgical instruments are heated, some viruses may still survive; no matter how antiseptic a surgical suite, you can always culture microbes off the floor. Despite the flushing of respirators or dialysis machines with powerful antiseptic solutions, and the use of the newest antibiotics, patients hooked to life-support machines still get infected. We can't get every mosquito either, or every tick that carries Rocky Mountain spotted fever. Vaccines are not available for all diseases, and even those we have may not be distributed properly and occasionally may even have unknown and potentially dangerous viruses growing in with the attenuated strains. Antitoxins, for all their effectiveness, are not always given soon enough, and many times are not available at all.

But if we did not have to be operated on, there would be no need to worry about sterile surgical suites. If water supplies are kept sterile and food uncontaminated, there is no need for the typhoid and cholera shots. If we didn't get infected, or suffered burns, then there would be no need for our antibiotics and antitoxins to be 100 percent effective. If our coronary arteries did not become clogged, we would not need to have coronary care units or bypass procedures. Treatments, no matter how sophisticated, are never the ultimate answer.

The only real answer for disease is prevention. This is especially true of cancer—not early diagnosis or even early treatment, but prevention. That is what the Surgeon General's Advisory Committee tried to do in its reports on the danger of cigarette smoking—protect us. It is what physicians have always tried to do, what has always given medicine its public value and individual worth.

The last great period when warnings in regard to public health were given occurred in connection with the infectious diseases. Between 1870 and 1910 over a hundred different infecting bacteria and well over thirty different disease-causing viruses and rickettsial parasites were discovered and the information distributed world-wide. In one twenty-year period alone, from 1872 to 1892, physicians and scientists isolated forty-five different microbes.

In 1874 Hansen described for the first time the bacillus of leprosy, and Neisser in 1879 the gonococcus, which causes gonorrhea. In 1880 Pasteur isolated the cholera bacillus, and Everth the bacillus causing typhoid fever. In 1881 Ogston described the staphylococcus, and the following year Rehleisen isolated the diphtheria microbe. In 1885 the tetanus organism was found. In 1887 Weichselbaum discovered the microbe that causes meningitis. In 1892 Pfeiffer isolated the influenza organism. In 1896 Exmergen described the cause of botulism, and Singer isolated the first variety of dysentery bacilli. Within a few years the actinomyces and nocardia fungi were discovered. Salmonella, brucellosis, pneumococcus, typhus, the Flexner bacillus, the *Haemophilus* organism *E. coli*, klebsiella, the *Serratia* group, *Aerobacter*, the *Mycoplasma*, scrub typhus, the cryptococcus, the syphilitic spirochete, the leptospire and the tularemia parasite were found. Then came the viruses: the adenoviruses, respiratory syncytial and yellow fever, the measles organism, mumps and chicken pox, the herpes simplex virus, herpes zoster, hepatitis A and B, cytomegalic-inclusion virus, and the virus that causes cat-scratch fever.

Even though all these discoveries involved causes of disease, not treatments, even though people were only being told what was killing them, the world still applauded each new discovery. There was no confusion, no cries of "Enough!" Indeed each new observation, each new fact, no matter how specific or limited, was met with almost instantaneous acceptance, with both success and fame for the discoverer. Pfeiffer, the man who isolated the influenza organism—offering no cures, no magic, not even hope to those infected—became known and honored throughout the world. Others were given titles and honorary degrees for discoveries, and men who did no more than simply develop the dyes to stain microbes became full professors of microbiology.

Yet today, physicians and scientists following in these men's footsteps, doing not only what they did, but more, not only discovering the causes of disease but at the same time offering the cures, are often met with outright ridicule. Even with the discovery in the eighteen-nineties of a whole new host of infecting organisms—the fungi—no one said, "My God, more damn infecting microbes." Even when by the nineteen-thirties we were deluged with a seemingly never-ending supply of at least five new microbial causes of human misery a year, no one ever cried "Enough! Why don't they just stop?" But this is exactly what is being said today. The new killers, the new cripplers of children and adults are being discovered now, not at the stunning rates with which infecting microbes were found, but in ones and twos, yet few seem to be listening. Indeed, each new discovery is met not only with disbelief but suspicion, and at times with open hostility.

The Surgeon General's Advisory Committee was created in 1961, yet after seven different publications about the dangers of cigarette smoking, spanning more than a decade, we are faced today with the same issue that brought the committee into existence—the rising death rate from lung cancer. Doing exactly what the infectious-disease experts of the nineteenth and early-twentieth centuries did, only better, the cancer researchers are not honored or even considered benefactors. Instead they are harassed and attacked, called charletans and manipulators of statistics.

These cancer scientists and physicians are portrayed by today's vested interests as suspect, as meddlers and troublemakers, but in the great tradition of medicine, in the struggle to continue to give medicine its value, they persevere. There are no rewards for what they accomplish, no Nobel prizes have been given out for studies of environmental carcinogenicity. Virtually no physician or medical student knows the names Rous and Berenblum. Unlike the case of the scientists and physicians who discovered the causes of infection to be staph and strep, the new discoveries about the causes of cancer bring not fame or fortune, but the risk of dismissal, loss of position and lack of advancement.

Even at the beginning of our understanding of infectious plagues there were those who tried to interfere, to deny the facts and subvert the truth.

The English physician John Snow, after a meticulous study of the cholera epidemics that intermittently ravaged the people of London, showed in 1854 that the disease was spread by polluted water. He presented his data, statistical in nature, tracing the spread of the disease along the water routes and drinking sources of the Thames. His data were attacked even to the point of his detractors' going down to the Thames and drinking from the river to prove to the public that English water could not carry disease.

But drinking the water didn't stop the plague any more than did the attacking of Snow's data. The cholera continued, and being an infectious disease, its time course was so rapid, so instantaneous that it was impossible to ignore. Parents seeing their children alive one day and watching them die the next, relatives burying one member of their family only to come home to find others doubled over with fever and cramps, were willing to try anything, and eventually refused to drink the river water. Relying on Snow's "statistical" data and heeding his warning, they put up with the inconvenience and added expense of bringing in water from the country. They closed the Broadstreet pump, and with that ended the plague, not just for that year but for every year thereafter.

Snow's data were accepted by the people in part because cholera, like all infectious diseases, was too devastating, too manifestly grotesque, too self-evident to be ignored. The self-interest of the public proved greater than the prejudices of those who, for whatever reason, saw no reason to act on the physician's warning. But a death is a death, whether infectious or not, an epidemic is an epidemic, and all of us are now in the midst of one as deadly as Snow's cholera.

A few people always survive an infectious disease. Not everyone in London was killed by cholera, nor today in the United States is 100 percent of the population stricken by influenza. Not everyone who contracts encephalitis dies from it. Even without treatment our bodies, because of different inocula of the infecting organisms, different avenues of microbial attack, past exposures as well as individual variations in immune responses, will always survive.

But virtually no one survives lung cancer, or angiosarcoma of the liver, mesotheliomas, or cancer of the pancreas. All the studies indicate that the great majority of such malignant cancers are environmentally induced. The only cure for them is

prevention, the elimination from the environment of the carcinogenic materials that cause them, so that we are no longer
exposed, so that our cells do not come in contact with even the
tiniest amounts of these cancer-inducing substances.

2.

Scientists have given us an important cue—a definitive diagnostic test—to determine what is a carcinogenic chemical and
what is not. Indeed, the development of this test is potentially
one of the most important environmental advances in modern-
day preventive medicine, and could in time be to cancer prevention what the development of the vaccines were to infectious diseases.

In an example of individual persistence combined with
scientific ingenuity and human concern, one man, Dr. Bruce
Ames of the University of California at Berkeley, did what
everyone said could not be done: he developed a test to prove
if a chemical could cause cancer. If, as he realized along with
other scientists, the majority of human cancers are caused
directly or indirectly by substances in the environment, what
was needed was a quick, reliable and inexpensive way of identifying the chemicals involved.

In Ames's own words: "About ten years ago I got fed up
reading the long list of chemicals on potato chip labels and
wondering if they were safe. . . . No one was testing anything
to see if there was a mutagen. . . . At any time something could
creep into our diet that would significantly alter our genes and
we would never know it. So I started manipulating bacteria to
see if I could sensitize them to detecting chemicals that can
cause mutations."

It took Ames a decade to develop his test. Since carcinogens
are mutagens, he reasoned that if a chemical caused a cell to

mutate, it would in all probability cause other cells to become malignant. All he needed was a way to look for cellular mutations, and he found one.

The test Ames finally devised is basically very simple. He developed a strain of bacteria that cannot grow in a certain type of nutrient-deficient broth, one without an amino acid called histidine, but can, with a slight change in its DNA—a mutation—begin to use the broth to grow.

The use of bacteria was just a convenient way to study the effects of chemicals on genetic material. Since all DNA, whether it comes from a microorganism, a mouse or a man, is basically the same, a chemical that damaged the DNA in the nucleus of a bacterium would in all probability damage the DNA in man. Bacteria are single-cell organisms. Like all living things, the nucleoprotein in their nucleus is chemically similar to the DNA in all other living things, including the DNA of our own cells.

The Ames test begins with the addition of small nontoxic amounts of the chemical under investigation to the special histidine-deficient broth. If the chemical gets into the bacterial cell, into the nucleus, and affects the bacteria's nucleoproteins, it will cause mutations and with the mutations some of the bacteria will begin to grow.

The Ames test system consists of a small covered laboratory dish filled with broth-growth medium seeded with millions of bacteria called *Salmonella typhimurium*. Ames has modified his bacterial strain genetically by selective breeding so that they cannot grow without histidine in the broth medium. The chemical to be tested is spotted on the broth, and the dish incubated at 37 degrees centigrade. At the end of two days the number of bacterial colonies that grow in the vicinity of the spots of the chemical are counted. The test is that simple and that definitive.

Each colony of growing bacteria represents a salmonella that has mutated, one that the test chemical has entered, changing its DNA, so that under new control the bacterial cell can now manufacture its own histidine, and unlike its unmutated neighbor not exposed to the spots of chemical, grow and divide in the histidine-different medium. The more colonies growing in the dish, the more active the chemical in causing mutation.

Ames continued to add variations to his test to make the system more applicable to humans. He peeled off the cell walls around the bacteria that ordinarily keep out large molecules. This has made the test sensitive to chemicals that might otherwise not be able to get into the bacteria. He has also incorporated liver enzymes into the culture medium, which can convert certain inactive test chemicals into active mutagens mimicking what happens to chemicals entering the human body, finding carcinogens forming from chemicals that by themselves, out in the environment and not yet ingested, might not be dangerous.

As a member of the National Institute of Environmental Health Sciences said recently: "This test system has proved its capability of identifying potentially dangerous chemicals in a quick and efficient way."

Benzopyrene has proved, as would be expected, to be mutagenic in the Ames bacterial system, as have aniline dyes and radiation. What happens to bacteria exposed to carcinogens is what happens to human cells. A gene in the cell's nucleus is injured. Like the mutated salmonella that can then grow in histidine-deficient broth, the genetically damaged human cell, its controls changed, short-circuited or suppressed, takes off in a new direction. Only unlike the mutated salmonella of the Ames test, not just to be able to use a deficient broth to grow, but to cause cancer.

That is really what cancer is. For all the suffering it causes, it is nothing more than a loss of intracellular control, a genetic mutation induced by injury. We tend to think of mutations in terms of the whole person, the albino or the dwarf, but the basis of all overt observable mutations is cellular.

If a mutation—damage to the nuclear DNA—occurs to embryonic cells during fetal development, the results show up as fetal deaths or congenital defects. If the mutation occurs in a fully matured cell, one that will not give rise to any other cell types, only that cell's nucleoprotein will be altered. But the change is still as permanent as any mutation in a fetal cell and will be passed on to all the cells that spring from it. Once DNA is changed, once the genetic code is altered, that change is permanent, forever.

It is held by some experts that cancer is the return of the malignantly transformed cell to a more primitive state, a state of earlier evolutionary development when it was less differentiated, less controlled than it was before its carcinogenic exposure and mutation. Mutations in matured cells are not advantageous. Anarchy is always right below the thin surface of control, whether in a biological system or in a civilization.

The effort in cellular evolution has always been toward greater order and control; more and more genes have continually been added to handle the ever more complicated cellular tasks. It is this control that has allowed multicellular life with all its interconnecting complexity to develop, and it is where the greatest amount of evolutionary energy has always been directed. If that control is interfered with or disrupted in any way, there is chaos. In the cities, the result is riot and anarchy; in our bodies, it is cancer.

We have now begun to realize that the problem of environmentally induced cancer is that the changes that are caused by the carcinogen are all internal, occurring in the cells' DNA; the surface of these malignant cells stay basically the same as normal cells'. There are essentially no new markers—no biologically active "antigens"—on their surface to be read as foreign by the body's defense system. Antigenetically like any other cells, ignored by the body's defense system, these malignant cells grow unrestricted, uncontrolled by any of our body's defense or reparative systems. That is why there is virtually no hope of survival for those who have smoking-induced lung cancer or asbestos-induced mesotheliomas.

3.

Ames has given us a test, a first step in making sure we are not exposed to carcinogenic substances. Food samples are tested all the time for bacterial contamination; no one thinks anything of it. Indeed, there is a great governmental bureaucracy devoted solely to the testing for bacterial contamination not only of foodstuffs but of water supplies. Public health, state health departments, city and municipal health officials, the Center for Disease Control in Atlanta, all are devoted to the control and prevention of communicable diseases. Bacterial or virally contaminated products when found are removed from the market or destroyed. Infected municipal water supplies are closed down. Companies that distribute salmonella- or botulism-contaminated products are allowed by a suspicious public to go bankrupt or lose substantial parts of their market, and everyone feels the loss is justified.

At a recent New York Academy of Science workshop, Dr. Fred de Serres said the Ames test "would help industry establish priorities on which chemicals to develop, allowing industry to screen chemicals very early in development instead of investing hundreds of thousands of dollars in a substance only to find out later it causes cancer."

With the use of the Ames test, in a matter of two days at a cost of approximately $600, rather than hundreds of thousands of dollars, the two to three years and the huge facilities necessary to do the appropriate animal studies, a potentially dangerous chemical can now be quickly screened for its ability to cause mutation, to damage the genetic material of cells.

There are industries today that resist the idea that their products may cause disease, just as in a former day the idea that illness could be caused by contaminated water was resisted. Recently Dr. Ames felt it necessary to write an open letter to Dr. John Menkart of the Clairol Corporation in response to a letter Menkart had sent out under Clairol's letterhead challenging not only Ames's conclusions about the carcinogenicity of hair-spray products but the validity of the test itself.

"I believe Menkart's letter is extremely misleading and irresponsible," Ames wrote. "We have developed a rapid and sensitive test using bacteria and animal tissue, for identifying mutagens, chemicals that damage the genetic material. Data obtained with this test have shown that over 80% out of 140 carcinogens tested show mutagenic activity while very few chemicals in general [100 noncarcinogens] are mutagenic. From the data we concluded that chemicals active in this test have a high probability of proving to be carcinogens. We find that 150 out of 169 oxidative-type hair dyes tested, most of the semi-permanent type dyes tested, nine of the components of hair dyes and several oxidation products of hair dye ingredients are mutagenic. Hair dye components can be absorbed apparently through the human scalp."

Others too have been concerned about the dangers of hair dyes but they, for whatever reasons, kept the dangers secret. *The F.D.A. Consumer* had stated even before Ames's letter that hair dyes "were specially exempted from the Federal

Food, Drug and Cosmetic Act of 1938 by Congress after
Industry persuasively argued that the dyes could not meet
safety standards of the act but should nonetheless be sold to
meet popular demands."

The fact is that the hair-dye industry had already guessed
wrong once about the dangers of their chemicals. 2, 4-
Diaminotoluene, which was used in hair dyes for many years,
was first shown to be a carcinogen in animal studies in 1955,
and again in 1969. Yet hair dyes containing this chemical were
still on the market as late as 1971.

What Ames had felt compelled to write about was not rates
of bacterial mutation, or the reproducibility of his results, but
human cancer and birth defects. Once a quiet cloistered
academician, he has had to do what concerned physicians and
scientists making discoveries opposed by vested interests have
always had to do. Like Snow more than a hundred years before
him, and Paracelsus and Paré centuries before Snow, Ames has
had to make a public fight for the public's health.

Like other courageous physicians and scientists before him,
Ames realized that the risks of keeping silent were too great,
the fabrications of those attacking his work too dangerous, for
him not to reply. It was the same with Semmelweis trying to
warn about the infectious nature of dirty hands. Only now it
is chemicals and carcinogens that the battle was about, not
bacteria.

X

The Perils of Radiation

1.

Radiation, more than any other environmental poison, has been life's oldest as well as its greatest enemy. Indeed, life has never been able to survive it. So devastating are the effects of radiation on living tissue that when life itself was being born it could not be assembled on the surface of the earth, or even near the surface, but only in the oceans at depths of from ten to twenty feet. Shielded by those three to five meters of water, the first cells could be formed while the oceans' surface, unprotected, was kept barren by the high-energy radiation pouring down from the sun. Cosmic rays and X-rays, like a deadly rain, swept clean the surface of the oceans and newly formed continents, leaving them barren. For two billion years those first cells, swaying back and forth in the seas' deep eddies, were sickened if they entered the murky twilight zones barely touched by visible light, and then, if they rose too near the surface, they were destroyed.

What happened to those first cells is what happened to the thyroid cells of the infants whose necks were irradiated, and to the bone-marrow cells of the radium workers, and to the people who died of radiation poisoning following the detonation of the atom bombs over Hiroshima and Nagasaki. The cells began to mutate, and then, with more exposures and more mutations, they died.

As those first primitive cells grew nearer the oceans' surface, the degree of radiation churning the waters around them continually increased. With less and less water to absorb the ionizing radiation, more and more rays penetrated their walls, and passing through their cytoplasm, collided with the DNA in their nuclei, at first causing simple mutations and later a loss of so much cellular control that cells took on bizarre shapes and even more bizarre actions, and finally, with more genetic injury, death.

Chemicals that are carcinogens or mutagens act by combining, destroying or interfering with the cells' DNA. It is the same with ionizing radiation. The ionizing rays are like tiny high-energy bullets. When they hit something, they destroy or disrupt what they hit. The linkages that hold together the molecules of DNA are still, as they always have been, uniquely susceptible to these rays.

Molecules, no matter how complex or intricate, are held together by minute, though measurable electronic linkages between the atoms that comprise them.. These linkages are incredibly small, and while still very strong, are really no more than shared electrons. Despite life's seeming durability, what binds it all together are these electrical linkages, connections that can be destroyed by high-energy fields. Forged when the earth was being formed, these bindings, the cement of the original polymers, the first enzymes—the shared electronic linkages that held together the sugars, phosphates and bases of the first DNA nucleoproteins and still hold them together— comprise a microscopic world of quantum force fields and electrostatic forces, some no more than one one trillionth of a volt, that are easily disrupted; the linkages quickly destroyed if hit by the high-energy ray of ionizing radiation.

A cell bombarded by a rain of high-energy radiation will eventually have one of those rays penetrate through to its nucleus, where it will hit a molecule of DNA and destroy the linkage holding together that part of the molecule. It is all very physical, like the shorting out of a toaster or the burning up of an overloaded transformer. If the injury is slight, perhaps the code for only one gene will be injured, but such is the economy of life that this one injury, this one broken linkage, will lead forever to an abnormal gene. A base may shift out of place, a sugar may be lost—whatever, the code will be altered and a genetic mutation will result.

In a sense, radiation was partly responsible for driving early evolution. As the first evolving cells, rising toward the oceans' surface, became subject to more and more radiation, they at first mutated; cells that were green became red, cells that could only use iron oxide for energy began to use hydrogen sulfide. As the radiation increased, though, more and more genes were injured. Eventually a gene controlling the synthesis of a cell's wall, or one cell's own metabolism, was injured, and then, without adequate support or transfer of energy, the cell died.

What finally did allow life to move to the surface of the oceans, and from there in an evolutionary explosion of cellular diversity onto the land and into the air, was the protection from radiation afforded by the production of oxygen following the evolutionary development of the first photosynthetic cells. Life's evolution had proceeded for millions of years where it began, in the oceans' depths. Eventually, under the pressure of increasingly scarce food supplies, photosynthetic cells emerged and with them the first production of oxygen.

Photosynethic cells could make their own food. They had evolved the internal ability to make sugars out of carbon dioxide and water. Oxygen was no more than the waste product of this reaction. Photosynthetic cells with their chemical ability to manufacture their own foods from the limitless surrounding supplies of carbon dioxide, water and the sunlight filtering down from the seas' surface became the dominant cell type in the evolving oceans. The molecules of oxygen discharged as waste products accumulated in the seas around them and then began eventually to diffuse out of the warm waters into the atmosphere surrounding the earth. The photosynthetic cells continued to grow and multiply, and over millions of years the amount of oxygen produced became staggering. The atmospheric level of oxygen slowly but gradually increased, and as it increased, the layers of oxygen absorbed more and more of the radiation raining down on the earth.

Produced by the action of cosmic rays on the atoms of oxygen, molecules of ozone began to be formed in the top layers of the newly developing atmosphere. The ozone absorbed even more of the radiation until cells, now having an atmosphere of protective oxygen and ozone to shield them and no longer needing the layers of water to protect them from the deadly rays, were able to rise to the oceans' surface. Populating what had been a sterile zone, they rapidly filled the oceans, and then the land, and eventually the sky.

2.

That cosmic radiation has not ended; it is still out there as it always has been, still raining down out of space onto the earth, held off from reaching us by nothing more than the atoms of oxygen and layer of protective ozone encircling the globe. If that atmosphere of oxygen or ozone is reduced in depth, the poisoned rain will reach us again.

At first only the cells of our skin will be damaged. Bombarded by the increased rain of radiation, the DNA of a few of these cells' nuclei will eventually be hit and sooner or later damaged. Genetic controls will be short-circuited, and the cell, reverting to a more primitive, less organized state, will eventually become overtly malignant. Day and night, radiation that had once been absorbed a hundred miles up will reach the earth's surface.

The National Research Council has calculated that a 10 percent decrease in the ozone of the atmosphere would permit enough excess ultraviolet radiation to reach the earth's surface to raise the incidence of skin cancer by 20 percent or more. With a further decrease in the ozone layer, more radiation will be let through, only now the rays, increased in intensity, will begin to pass through our skin and hit the nuclei of the cells lying deeper in our bodies, and finally, with an even greater increase in the bombardment, the genes in the nuclei of our own sperm and eggs. Unheard and unfelt, the radiation will eventually cause all kinds of cancers, and then through mutations, the end of life itself.

It is not a foolish or far-fetched concern; radiation-induced destruction of life happened not only at the beginning of the world, but probably has occurred cyclically at other times since then. In a paper published in *Nature*, G. C. Reid and I. S. A. Isaksen, both of the National Oceanic and Atmospheric Administration, and T. E. Hulzer and Paul Crutzen of the National Center for Atmospheric Research suggested that solar high-energy particles regularly wreak havoc on life during the periodic reversals of the earth's magnetic fields that deplete the ozone layer and let in the increasing and lethal doses of ultraviolet radiation.

These scientists postulate that such deadly periodic bombardment could well explain the sudden disappearance through the earth's history of many animals and plant species from the single-cell ocean-dwelling organisms to the dinosaurs. The danger is still there. The threat to ourselves and our children's future is where it has always been—behind the clouds.

A large part of the controversy over supersonic aircraft arises from concern about their effects on the ozone layer. Laboratory tests and chemical theory have shown that the nitrogen oxides given off by jet engines destroy ozone. The argument that all this is simply theory based on restricted laboratory conditions no longer holds. The same effects of oxides have been shown to occur in the stratosphere itself.

The dangerous cosmic radiation was never disposed of but simply absorbed by the earth's atmosphere, held off from endangering life by a layer of ozone no more than a quarter mile thick. Radiation in any form is so destructive to cellular life that, cosmic or atomic, diagnostic or therapeutic, the only protection from it is prevention.

It is estimated that a fleet of SST's—supersonic transports of the type considered for development in the United States and already in operation by the British and French, could cause a 10 percent reduction in ozone over the northern hemisphere alone.

The same reduction can occur from aerosol containers freeing gases into the atmosphere, aerosols serving no other purpose than a kind of foolish convenience, a convenience easily replaced by atomizers and hand-operated sprays.

The sky with its canopy of oxygen and ozone protects each of us as the depths of the oceans' waters once protected the beginning of life; and with some effort and common sense that protection can continue.

The Du Pont company, the manufacturer of a component of aerosol container, apparently agrees, but only in the text of scientific journals, not in their advertisements. In a series of letters reminiscent of what Ames had to face with the Clairol

Corporation, F. S. Rowland and Mario J. Molena, two of the scientists who first called attention to the dangers of ozone depletion, felt obliged to attack a Du Pont advertisement which had appeared in several newspapers and magazines. The advertisement stated: "The ozone depletion theory, based on a computer model of the stratosphere, was reported in 1974 by two chemists at the University of California. . . . In order to estimate hypothetical reactions and because little is actually known about real ones, the modelers made a number of assumptions about the way the atmosphere behaves."

In their own letter to Du Pont published in *Science*, the two scientists wrote: "The statements about our assumptions were not made by us, but are apparently inferences drawn by the writers of the advertisement." Listing where their data had been published, definitively giving additional scientific references that supported and substantiated their work, they concluded: "[Our] concern is with *changes* from the natural situation caused by man. Our original conclusion was that, at current rates of technological use, fluorocarbons 11 and 12 [components of aerosols] were the two most important man-made compounds, in terms of potential effects on the ozone layer. This conclusion still stands, and has been amplified and supported by numerous studies, including direct stratospheric experiments. We believe that sufficient facts are already available in the refereed scientific literature to establish that chlorine released by stratospheric photolysis of fluorocarbons 11 and 12 will indeed have a substantial effect on the average ozone level of the earth in the future if present usages are maintained."

Rowland and Molena's letter was sent by the editors of *Science* to the E. I. Du Pont de Nemours Company. The company's answer, reprinted in *Science*, began: "Du Pont's advertisement was not intended to attack the published scientific work of Rowland and Molena on ozone depletion, which, we have said before, we believe to have raised a significant point.

"The principal source of misunderstanding appears to be that the authors interpret the advertisement to say they made certain assumptions in their 'actual experiments.' To the contrary, the assumptions lie in the products of their research— particularly in the public position taken by Rowland with regard to the implications of their research."

In other words, Du Pont did not question Rowland and Molena's scientific data, but objected to their making the data public.

Yet, what worried Rowland and Molena about the atmosphere is happening right now beneath the ozone canopy. It is what is happening here on earth that is our greatest immediate threat. We still have the atmosphere between us and the constant flood of lethal cosmic radiation. But we have no protective shield between us and our machines, no layers of ozone and oxygen, no ten to twelve feet of ocean water to shield us from them.

3.

Within seconds after the atom bomb was dropped on Hiroshima, thousands were killed where they stood. Those who were not blown apart were burned to death by the heat from the fireball. Pieces of rock and flying glass decapitated children, parts of falling buildings cut off arms and legs, splinters of ricocheting bricks and mortar were driven into hearts and brains, arteries were severed and veins torn. Those wounded who were not killed instantly soon bled to death and died where they lay.

The survivors of the initial blast thought, when they had buried their loved ones and begun to clean up their city, all that remained for them was their grief and heartache. They were wrong. When the rubble was finally cleared, the dead and pieces of the dead buried, when those who had survived the original detonation but were left crippled and mutilated were finally beginning to put their lives together, the second deaths began.

They started slowly, perniciously, with a little vomiting and some diarrhea. Within weeks, men and women who thought they had escaped the fiery holocaust started losing weight and began to notice that their hair was falling out. When finally, too weak and exhausted to work, they went to their doctors, strange anemias were diagnosed.

Then the infections began, the pneumonias, and the meningitises, the abscesses and the boils. Survivors watched horrified while members of their families and their friends, seemingly untouched by the bomb, people they had thanked God were still with them, still alive, screamed out in the middle of the night and began vomiting blood. Children who just days before had looked well began to double over in pain and bleed from the nose and mouth.

The dying began again. Those who thought they were done with the sufferings began to realize there was something more to the detonation of that bomb than just the heat and the blast. Within months, thousands more were dead. Radiation poisoning killed almost as many people as those who had died in the original heat and blast.

Yet those who survived the radiation poisoning and still remained alive were not yet done with the dying. In truth, death was always to be the survivors' lot. The terrible march which began in that one brilliant millisecond of nuclear fusion would go on and on. Within two years after the burial of the last person with radiation poisoning, the leukemias and bone cancers began.

Those who had survived the immediate blast and were far enough away from the epicenter of the bomb's detonation to escape the flying bricks and the heat, the killing dosages of radiation, thought surely now the horrors were over. But they were mistaken. Men who had made Herculean efforts to put their lives and their cities back together again began to have chest pain, have trouble moving and even sleeping, and were told they had bone cancer. Women, feeling dizzy, who had already buried their sons and husbands, were told by their doctors they had leukemia.

The horrors were never to end. As in a Kafka novel, those who continued to survive continued to be punished. Even now, thirty years later, what began in the blast and the noise still goes on. Children who were not killed in the first few seconds after the blast, who did not die later from the radiation, leukemia or bone cancers, just died.

Experimental evidence has shown clearly that exposure to ionizing radiation shortens the life span of animals. The report on the human effects of radiation following the blast at Nagasaki clearly states, "there is a higher neonatal (newborn) and infant mortality within 2000 meters of the epicenter unrelated to parental age, birth order, third trimester, or socioeconomic class." In short, within a mile of the blast infants simply died—no cause.

It was not as if we didn't know about the genetic effects of radiation. The scientists who developed the A-bomb and the officials who ordered it to be dropped knew of the dangers. Experimental work done in the 1920's and 1930's had clearly shown the terrible genetic effects that could be caused by radiation, the extraordinary susceptibility of fetal tissues to radiation's damaging effects, and the dangers of cancer production. Not only is radiation carcinogenic, specifically damaging to the DNA of mature cells, but experiment after experiment had shown that pregnant animals exposed to radiation in any form, even though unharmed themselves, gave birth to grossly deformed fetuses. The issue was again poisoning from an environmental toxin, in this case a physical rather than a chemical one, but the results were the same.

In 1952, in an article entitled "Radiation Hazards to the Embryo and Fetus," published in the *Journal of Radiology*—and supported by the Atomic Energy Commission itself—L. B. Russel, of the Biology Division of the Oak Ridge Laboratory in Tennessee, wrote: "The developing embryo of a great variety of animal forms studied, including several mammals, is highly susceptible to the induction of malformations by radiation. There is no reason to doubt that this also applies to human embryos. Animal experiments have clearly demonstrated that there are well-defined critical periods in the development of most characteristics. That is, a particular abnormality may be produced by irradiation at a particular stage or stages but not at all from irradiation at other stages. Critical periods in man correspond to the second to sixth week of gestation. During at least part of this period pregnancy may be unsuspected. . . . Dosages high enough to produce developmental abnormalities do not necessarily cause abortions or prenatal deaths [while nevertheless, by injuring the DNA of the fetal cells, producing severe congenital abnormalities]. Irradiation at more advanced stages of fetal development [more mature, more differentiated cells] produce less obvious and possibly more delayed effects which from the human point of view may be as harmful as the gross monstrosities—defects such as cataracts, malformed eyes and microcephaly, as well as brain damage, mental retardation, spinal cord injuries, delayed growth and development, and suppression of antibody function."

Injure the DNA of a fetal cell at any time, in any way, and

the result is cellular chaos. Pregnant animals exposed to experimental radiation had been born with twisted heads and malformed skeletons long before atomic power was even dreamed of. The radium workers were dying of their leukemias and bone cancers even as the first nuclear pile was being constructed. The hands of the first fluoroscopists had already become no more than cancerous stumps when Fermi and Oppenheimer began assembling the bomb.

4.

Notwithstanding all we know about the peril of radiation, we have continually underestimated its dangers and have always paid the price for that misunderstanding. In the first days of isotopic research, even after we knew all about the radium workers, the effects of radiation on fetal cells, the destroyed hands of the first fluoroscopists, even after the bomb had been dropped and thousands had already died from radiation poisoning, even while others there at Hiroshima and Nagasaki were beginning to develop their cancers, five hundred patients were injected with radioactive plutonium as part of a medical research experiment. Two hundred of those injected went on to develop liver cancer and die.

In Japan there is a saying: "Many people mistake Hiroshima for yesterday; it is really tomorrow." For those two hundred people that tomorrow had arrived. The scientists, not knowing enough and underestimating the effects of what they considered a safe dose of a safe isotope, signed the death warrants for almost half their patients by injecting the isotope.

The report entitled "The Effects on Populations of Exposure to Low Levels of Ionizing Radiation," published by the Advisory Committee on the Biological Effects of Ionizing

Radiations, of the National Academy of Science; the report of the Adrian Committee of England; the Oxford Study of Childhood Cancer; the article on "Radiation Hazards to the Embryo and Fetus," in the *Journal of Radiology;* and hundreds more just like them published over half a century of research and study have bit by bit laid the scientific groundwork for the real concerns about radiation, concerns that have nothing to do with the catastrophe of a nuclear detonation. There is not a word in any one of these reports about bodies blown apart or fireballs. Instead they talk about the less dramatic but more lasting and more terrifying aspects of radiation exposure.

In 1956 Alice Stewart, in a retrospective study of children with malignancies, showed that the rate of exposure in utero (exposures of a child while still being carried by the mother) to diagnostic X-rays was about 50 percent higher for children with malignancies than for controls. It was a preliminary report, but as Dr. Stewart stated in her article: "Public Health officials all over the country are engaged in an environmental survey which will eventually cover 1,500 children who died of leukemia or malignant disease before the age of ten from the year 1953–55. As yet only approximately a third of the case material has been gathered, but preliminary analysis has yielded a result which should, we feel, be reported without further delay."

She went on to state: "The following facts have been known for a long time: First, excess exposure to radioactive materials leads not only to immediate radiation sickness and death, but to the development of leukemia and cancer. Second, the immediate ill effects of radiation are disproportionally great when the whole body is exposed; thirdly, therapeutic radiation of pregnant women is able to cause microcephaly and other congenital defects in the fetus.

"To this we must now add that radiotherapy can cause

cancer in children. Our study suggests that besides causing genetic damage, this apparently harmless examination [X-rays of pregnant women] may occasionally cause leukemia or cancer in the child [years after birth]."

It was radiation to the thymus all over again; only now it was not cancer of the thyroid at twenty and thirty years after irradiation, but leukemia at five and ten years, and now it wasn't adults who were dying, but children. One experimental study after another had shown the incredible sensitivity of fetal tissues to ionizing radiation. Now it was proved for humans. Nothing has changed; fetal cells adrift in tides and currents of the mother's body are today at the same risk of injury from ionizing radiation as their ancestors were while rising and falling in the drifts of the first seas.

In an article entitled "Investigation of the Effects of Prenatal X-Ray Exposure of Human Oogonia and Oocytes [human eggs] as Measured by Later Reproductive Performance," published in the *American Journal of Epidemiology*, Meyers, the author, wrote: "Many factors influence the response of living cells to ionizing radiation. Mammalian cells are generally more susceptible than insect cells. Within an individual some tissues are altered or destroyed by lower [amounts of] radiation than others. . . . Sperm cells are destroyed by low doses of radiation. The few that survive will eventually recover [and repopulate the testes]. . . . This is not true with eggs. Animals exposed to radiation have defective eggs."

What Meyers goes on to explain in his article and to worry over is what every embryologist and even every medical student knows: sperm cells, made in the testes, are replaced each day, continually, but the eggs a female has in her ovaries are there from the time she is born; no new eggs are ever made again. When the fetal ovaries are developing inside an unfolding female embryo, a few cells already inside of that embryonic organ divide off and begin to form themselves into the eggs that she as an adult will carry all her life. After puberty, one of these eggs will be released each month for all of her reproductive life. There are estimates that the cortex of each woman's ovary contains approximately half a million eggs. There will always be enough eggs; nature has taken care of the numbers. But if those cells are injured at any time, even when the future mother herself is being formed, it is her children that will be injured—that will pay the price not for their own misfortune or for that of their mother's, but for their grandmother's mistake.

It has already been proved for second generations. A Danish researcher, Zachacer Christiansen, studied the outcome of pregnancies in women who had received X-ray exposures in the pelvic region for diseases of the pelvic bones and for hemangriomas. Among offspring of these women (who had been irriadated in areas that exposed their ovaries) the author observed an increased rate of absorption, fetal deaths and prematurity as compared with the whole population of Denmark for the equivalent years 1918–1958.

Even childhood X-ray exposures in cases of congenitally dislocated hips showed that female infants exposed to multiple diagnostic pelvic X-rays gave birth after they became sexually mature to offspring with a higher frequency of abnormalities and lower birth weights than controls.

The dangers, though, brought about by preceding generations' mistakes, which this next generation and the one even more removed may have to pay the price for, also involve drugs. The use of the drug Diethylstilbestrol (DES) in pregnant women confirmed in a terrible way for drugs what the diagnostic X-ray exposure studies had already proved, that pregnant mothers exposed to potential carcinogens may be dooming not themselves but their children to cancer.

A number of women in the late fifties and sixties were given DES to avoid the threat of miscarriage in early pregnancy. The drug entered their fetuses' circulation, interfering with the normal development of the embryonic vagina in the female fetuses these women were carrying. Structures that normally should have disappeared were retained. At puberty, when the girls were on the threshold of womanhood, cells in these abnormally retained structures, exposed for the first time to the developmental influences of the girls' own sex hormones, became cancerous. Instead of developing into a mature vaginal epithelium, these injured cells turned overtly malignant.

Researchers report that of the thousands of daughters born by women who took DES, as of April 1976 the drug was the cause of at least 120 fatal cancers.

5.

It is the same with other diseases.

In 1961 Irene Uchida showed that Mongolism, a devastating all-encompassing congenital defect caused by injured chromosomes, could be caused by irradiation. The genes that are damaged are not crucial to life and death, only to normal development. The fetus, even with its chromosomes damaged, continues to develop, but the damage occurring early in fetal development becomes widespread.

This cell doesn't form quite right; that cell produces the wrong enzyme. This tissue is structurally unsound; that one does not conduct properly. The child is born, but it is a disaster. That one microscopic chromosomal defect occurring early in development and passed on to each newly forming cell results in multiple congenital defects: a small head, heart defects, hernias, large tongue, abnormal joints, malformed ears, cataracts, abdominal distention, short stature and mental retardation. Mongoloids live like this, retarded, deformed all their lives—for fifty and sixty years.

Uchida in her study sent questionnaires to the parents of Mongoloid children, inquiring about any radiation the mothers might have received before the child was born. The mothers were divided into three groups: those who had received no abdominal X-rays, those with fewer than four exposures, and those with four or more. She found that a substantial number of the mothers of Mongoloids had been irradiated.

Nowhere in her study, indeed nowhere in any of the studies on the increased incidence of leukemias, stillborns and congenital malformations in children whose mothers were exposed to radiation, is there mention of an atomic blast. No one even mentions the vomiting or diarrhea of radiation poisoning, the pain of wasting away, the embarrassment of having one's hair fall out. The studies deal only with diagnostic levels of irradiation, and what they say quite simply is that as far as we can tell, there may well be no lower limit to the amounts of radiation or radioactivity a cell can tolerate.

The supplement to the controversial 1962 British Committee Report of "Radiologic Hazards to Patients" begins: "As far as genetic effects are concerned, it seems clear enough that any radiation exposure, however small, has a certain probability of causing point mutations in sperm cells." The supplement goes on to say, "Sufficient exposure to radiation is certainly leukemogenic in man," and concludes, "We can no longer content ourselves by saying that hazards from radiation like leukemia *may perhaps* be produced by relatively low levels of radiation damage."

More recently W. M. Court Brown, R. Poll and A. B. Hill, following 39,000 children irradiated in utero for diagnostic purposes, and concerned about the future development of cancer rather than of congenital defects, concluded that simple radiologic examination of the mother's abdomen similar to routine chest X-rays of males, during the early stage of pregnancy, raised the chances of the exposed child's developing leukemia in later life by as much as 50 percent. In 1957, physicians studying the incidence of leukemia in patients given deep X-ray therapy to the spine showed beyond any doubt the relationships between the dose of radiation received and the increasing incidence of what were pure radiation-induced malignancies. Article after article has forged a ring of irrefutable evidence which at the very minimum proves that irradiation of cells, and especially fetal cells, is carcinogenic in the widest sense of the word.

A paper published recently in the *World Health Organization Chronicle* entitled "Genetic Risks from Medical Radiation" put the whole concern about radiation exposure in perspective: "It has been known for a long time that irradiation of the skin may lead to cancer of the skin, irradiation of the bone marrow to leukemia, and irradiation of the thyroid to cancer of this organ. Whole-body irradiation or irradiation of major parts of the body may shorten the life span, and irradiation of the gonads creates genetic changes, in particular an increased mutation frequency, which may result in hereditary diseases or in a deterioration of the level of health in future generations."

All the effects mentioned above have one characteristic in common: "radiation increases the probability of their occurrence to an extent depending on the dose received."

It matters little or not at all where the radiation comes from —exposure from X-ray machines, atomic detonation, the sun, radioactive isotopes, abnormal discharges from nuclear power plants—they are all the same. Any radiation from any source can be dangerous. Many scientists agree with R. H. Mole, who

wrote in the *Journal of Nuclear Medicine*, "There is no a priori
reason why if mild dosages of radiation can produce leukemia
or cancer in moderate frequency small doses of radiation should
not do so in lower frequency."

In a society where scientists have the final word in almost
every technological decision, the overwhelming body of scientific evidence is that exposures to ionizing radiation, no matter
how small, are at the very least additive, and that while we can't
be sure at exactly what level of radiation exposure the DNA of
a cell can be injured, the sensible course is to keep all exposures
to the very minimum. This is what we do today, at least in
medicine.

The data showing the danger of exposing pregnant women
to irradiation, the studies uncompromisingly accepted by the
medical profession, are of exactly the same quality, the same
statistical nature, containing the same "probabilities," rather
than "real risks," as all the other environmental studies on
carcinogens challenged by the various industrial interests involved. Indeed, the risks from diagnostic irradiation of pregnant women are much less overall than the risks from cigarette
smoking or exposure to ultraviolet irradiation or even from
exposures to many of the other environmental carcinogens. Yet
physicians refuse to take even that small risk unless it is absolutely necessary. On the strength of "statistical data" they
refuse to submit pregnant women to unnecessary radiations of
any kind. So widespread is this understanding today that such
irradiation may very well be a cause for a malpractice suit.

It is important to realize why, from the very beginning, no
one challenged this ban on X-raying during pregnancy, why
there were no lobbies, no industry advertisements attacking the
nature of these studies. The reason for the acceptance of the
scientific facts of the dangers of irradiating pregnant women

is that there were no business interests involved with maintaining such exposures, no profit-and-loss statements to be derived from continuing the procedures. The only concern here was with health and protection, and as a result no physician today puts a pregnant woman in front of an X-ray machine and presses the button unless it is absolutely necessary.

Yet our government proposes to have three hundred nuclear power plants in operation throughout the country by 1990.

6.

The potential for human disaster is gigantic. The answer to the question of whether the small amounts of radiation discharged from nuclear power plants during normal operation or necessary maintenance procedures are dangerous, or will be dangerous after twenty and thirty years of constant discharging, is not yet known. What we do know is that the small scatter of radiation which eventually caused malignant transformations in the thyroids of infants exposed barely a generation ago has proved to be much more dangerous than expected.

The immediate problem concerning nuclear power is not whether the low levels of human exposure to the small amounts of radiation released from these plants during their daily operation will or will not prove ultimately harmful. What is critical is the question: Can we afford as a nation or as individuals to run the risk of exposing ourselves and our children to the unshielded radiation that could result from a plant disaster, a disaster involving nothing as sensational as a melt-down but only the possibility of safety cables being cut and compressors failing?

You would expect today's scientists to be in the forefront of those warning us about the dangers we face. In a world of ever more complex technology and expertise, it not only should be, but it can only be those directly concerned with the developing technologies, the theories and the hardware, those possessing full knowledge of what they are dealing with and what is being done, who can see the risks and the dangers, who must sound the warning.

Yet it is precisely those most qualified to warn us about our man-made dangers who are the most vulnerable, the most susceptible to economic and political pressures. Today it is the scientist who has the most to lose by speaking out. The very uniqueness of his training, the highly specialized nature of his knowledge and skills limits the opportunity for his employment. If you are a nuclear scientist involved with plasma flows and fission reactions, safety shields and sodium pumps, or a solid-state physicist involved with computer panels, there are only certain specific jobs available and those for the most part are limited to only a few large companies. It is not only the possibility of being fired, but of being blackballed by an entire industry, of not ever again being able to get a job in your speciality, that makes any public scientific statement about technical risks, dangers or deficiencies a very courageous affair. It has been like that for decades now, but especially in the field of nuclear energy.

With the splitting of the atom in the late thirties, scientists began thinking of using atoms for energy. World War II side-tracked their efforts, focusing scientific attention on the development of bombs rather than energy. When the war ended, the effort in atomic development was once again channeled into energy production. Gathering together the same enthusiastic drive that had led to the development of the bomb, the atomic scientists pushed on into reactors. Under the pressures for development and production, problems that couldn't be

solved or were too difficult to find adequate answers to were
simply shelved or patched over, the idea being that later, with
ever more technology and theoretical insights, solutions would
be found.

The greatest of these problems, as always with radiation, was
safety. This was the problem that most vexed the nuclear-
power-plant scientists, the problem they continually put off
and that in fact they never really found an adequate answer for.
Today that problem no longer faces just them, but us.

A major accident in a Consolidated Edison coal plant, an
explosion at a water-operated electrical generating plant, a
failure of a backup safety system at a fuel-oil-run operation can
be contained. The disaster can be restricted. This is not the
case with radioactivity. The issue now is what it has always
been—the very special and unique danger of radioactivity to
living cells and the terrible inability we have had in controlling
even small amounts of it.

Scientists connected with the government agency established to safeguard nuclear power plants (formerly the Atomic
Energy Commission, recently renamed the Nuclear Regulatory
Agency) admit that a significant leak of radioactivity from a
nuclear plant would at the very minimum lead to from between
40,000 and 80,000 cancer deaths among those exposed individuals in the areas surrounding the plant. One gram of
gaseous radioactive plutonium released into the atmosphere
would be enough to eventually cause lung cancer in virtually
every human being on earth. The land around a major plant
disaster would be unusable for hundreds if not thousands of
years. Any accident which would lead to an abnormal release
of radioactivity, a break in the safety containers around a reactor, a broken pipe, would cause any or all of this.

The incendiary raids on Tokyo and Dresden may have killed
more than the initial blast and heat from the A-bomb deto-

nated over Hiroshima and Nagasaki, but then the dying stopped. No one who survived lived only to die months later of radiation poisoning, or years later of leukemia and bone cancer. There was no increased incidence of fetal deaths and prematurity. The land could be used again; the dead could give way to the living.

The medical profession has listened to the Meyerses and the Uchidas and the Stewarts; we have accepted the dangers of radiation spelled out in the Adrian and Oxford reports. We no longer give radioactive iodine to pregnant women or irradiate thymuses. Yet, with the greatest nuclear power plant already working for us a safe 96 million miles away, with the ability tomorrow of cutting our use of energy by almost 50 percent without any noticeable decrease in our quality of life by simply elminating energy-wasteful procedures, by building better buildings and smaller cars, the government scientists and energy executives still push for more and more nuclear power plants, claiming as an excuse the need for more energy. It is interesting to note that we in the United States use more energy yearly just for air conditioning than China consumes in twelve months for all her needs.

The Brown Ferry Energy plant in Alabama was recently, according to some sources, within hours of a melt-down. A fire caused by a candle burned away both the main safety and backup cables controlling the reactor. Fortunately the plant officials were able to lower the pressure in the reactor in time so that other, less efficient pumps could be brought on line.

The Vermont Yankee nuclear power plant was recently closed because of the discovery of a potential flaw in its safety system that could have permitted a devastating nuclear accident. The discovered potential design flaw might have resulted in what both supporters and critics of nuclear power regard as the worst possible nuclear accident—a breakdown in the safety

container shielding the nuclear reactor—allowing the implo-
sion of both high-pressure steam and superheated water
through the barrier and the outward escape of radioactive
material.

Dr. Robert Pollard, a project manager for the Nuclear
Regulatory Agency, recently resigned because of his concern
over the nuclear power plant called Indian Point #3 being
built forty miles north of New York City. Three other scientists, working for General Electric, one of the nation's main
contractors for nuclear power plants, also resigned to speak out
against what they felt were not only inadequate safety procedures and obsolete machinery but measures and machinery
which, even working properly, would not be adequate for plant
protection.

Recently Ernst J. Effenberger, a senior engineer working
since 1972 on the planning stages for the world's first floating
nuclear power plant, felt obliged to resign to warn the three-
man Atomic Safety and Licensing Board of the Nuclear
Regulatory Commission about the folly of even trying to build
such a plant on the oceans.

The Rasmussen Report—a report undertaken by the federal
government "to estimate the public risks that could be involved in potential accidents in commercial nuclear power
plants of the type now in use" and especially "to make a
realistic estimate of these risks and, to provide perspective, to
compare them with non-nuclear risks to which our society and
its individuals are already exposed"—has stated that nuclear
power is as safe or safer than other ordinary risks of life.

Some, like Dr. Barry Commoner, have argued that the report's comparison of nuclear and non-nuclear risks is like comparing apples and oranges. "It seems to me," Dr. Commoner
writes, "there is no valid comparison between the risks of
personal tragic individual events like automobile accidents and

the risks of operating a device which has the acknowledged, designed capacity—however improbable—of killing tens of thousands of people."

The report has also been criticized for its assumptions; the fact that it does not consider the possibility of sabotage; its assumption of the efficient evacuation of surrounding populations. Attacks have also been leveled at the computer codes used to develop the report's predictions, and its neglect of the potential dangers in the nuclear fuel cycle itself—the reprocessing of nuclear fuel, its transportation as well as storage.

Dr. George Kistiakowsky, a Harvard physical chemist and explosives expert, has questioned the Rasmussen Report's assumption that most melt downs would not be catastrophic.

Charles F. Zimmermann and Robert O. Pohl of Cornell University have questioned the fact that in listing the different ways in which the equipment in a reactor could fail, the authors of the report decided not to study fires. In fact, according to Zimmermann and Pohl, the authors of the report made a "qualitative judgment" not to consider fires in their calculations. This is strange, Pohl writes, since fires have always been the major cause of damage at government-owned nuclear facilities.

Even Dr. Rasmussen himself has apparently questioned that reactors are as reliable as the report assumes. In 1974 he wrote in *Combustion:* "Probably one of the most serious issues that the intervenors [critics of nuclear power] can raise today, with good statistics to back their case, is that the nuclear power plants have not performed with the degree of reliability we would expect from machines built with the care and attention to safety and reliability that we have so often claimed."

Even if you believe in the need for nuclear power plants and that those scientists who are warning us about the dangers of nuclear power are being unreasonable, you are still faced with the problem of what to do with radioactive wastes. At the very minimum, if present plans for nuclear power are fulfilled, we will be putting the burden of lighting our homes and cities and running our machinery on our children. They will be the ones who will have to deal with the poisons we bequeath them.

The halflife of plutonium is 24,360 years, that of uranium over 4 million. There is as yet and probably never will be a safe place, a safe container, a safe storage area for radioactive wastes that can be maintained for an entire generation, much less a hundred or a thousand years. We will be endangering, in the most real way, our own children and our grandchildren, exposing them to cancer and fetal deaths, congenital defects and retardation by lining their world with our radioactive wastes.

There is a small town in Canada, near the American border, called Port Hope. In the thirties a plant was built in this town to process radium from pitchblende. In the forties the plant switched to refining uranium. During its ten years of pitchblende operation, 100,000 tons of radioactive rubble and garbage was generated by the plant's operation. Much was carted away, but some was used for landfills around the town. In those years, too, workers carried home from the plant discarded but still slightly radioactive building materials for home repairs. Beginning a year ago, a radiation spot check of the homes and schools surrounding the town revealed increased levels of radioactivity twenty to thirty times what is considered normal.

Ten years earlier, in the sixties, a family living near one of the town's schools noticed that the plants in their garden bordering the school lot never grew; even the trees they planted died. They were never able to grow anything in that soil. That school when checked for radioactivity was found to have such high radiation levels in the basement and lunchroom that the school had to be closed, and in all probability it will never be opened again.

The fill poured over twenty years earlier for the school's foundation was contaminated with radioactive wastes from the plant. Over the years the radium in the contaminated soil was slowly converted by the oxygen in the air to radon gas. A small amount of this highly radioactive gas had seeped through the school's foundation. This meant that twenty years' worth of children had been continually exposed eight hours a day, five days a week, to increased levels of radiation.

For a decade the water, too, draining from the dumps outside the city had carried radium down to within the city itself, contaminating the homes as the school had been. Parents have taken now to trying to keep their babies out of the basement playrooms while they worry about what might happen to their older children, those who had already been exposed, some for years.

But it doesn't end with Port Hope. Recently an oceanographer with the Environmental Protection Agency located and examined, for the first time, two ocean dumping areas used by the Atomic Energy Commission between the years 1946 and 1970 for the disposal of low-level nuclear wastes. He found evidence of contamination of the oceans caused by radioactive wastes leaking from these dump sites. Many of the 61,800 55-gallon drums making up the two disposal sites were found to be crushed. The oceanographer concluded that permeance of disposal had never been a consideration; that the purpose of sinking the barrels was simply to get rid of the wastes, and once out of sight, hopefully out of mind.

At the present time, wastes from commercial reactors are collected in underwater storage basins at the plant sites themselves. But the commercial storage basins are filling up, and soon after 1980 there will be little remaining space for wastes from reactors now operating. If permanent storage is not found elsewhere, the plants will have to close down. Today, the only two designated permanent "long-term" storage sites in the United States are for military wastes, one in Washington State and the other in South Carolina, and both of these are known to have already suffered leaks. There is really no place to put the wastes.

When the A-bomb was finally assembled in the winter of 1945, its two chief architects, Enrico Fermi and J. Robert Oppenheimer, had a decision to make. They had calculated that the chance that the detonation might ignite the whole atmosphere and kill all mankind was 3 in 1 million, but they decided to detonate it anyway. The bomb was exploded at Alamogordo in July 1945. The world survived.

Some of the young scientists and administrators who were present at the birth of the A-bomb, men who agreed with Fermi and Oppenheimer's decision, moved out of the New Mexico desert into government and into corporations, to administer commissions and help run the huge energy companies so intimately involved with developing atomic energy. Today, ignoring the dangers of nuclear power plants, the studies of radioactive exposures, they play down the concerns of other scientists. Those concerned, though, can simply no longer be ignored by scientists, laymen or physicians.

XI

Prevention
the Only Cure

The concern in all this is not death, but life. No one is asking for a moratorium on dying, only on the kind of senseless death that is going on all around us.

When a man like Bertrand Russell dies, simply of old age, we feel little need for mourning. Whatever our sense of loss, we know he had lived his life to the full, and there was even a certain correctness to his end.

This is not the feeling we have when we think of those adolescent girls who were killed by cancer of the vagina because their mothers while pregnant were given the drug Diethylstilbestrol during the early part of their pregnancies. Even years later there is still grief in the homes of these girls, still the sense of guilt we all feel for lives unfulfilled. The drug should have been destroyed a decade ago. Yet meat producers still want to add it to the diet of cows, to provide greater weight gain with less feed. The sad fact is that the use of DES as an additive for animal feeds is still under consideration by government regulatory agencies.

In the past hundred years we have managed to eliminate one scourge after another—cholera and rabies, typhus, typhoid, smallpox and yellow fever. There are no iron lungs being wheeled off planes any more, nor are there wards filled with retarded children whose brains have been ravaged by measles. The battle against the infectious diseases has largely been won.

Today we are faced with an entirely different kind of plague, where the enemy is no longer bacteria or viruses but man. Yet the principle involved in this battle is the same as that already won in the the struggle to cure the infectious diseases—prevention. The answer for polio was not a better iron lung, and the cure for cancer is not a more radical operative procedure. Prevention is the only answer.

We are not doomed to die of cancer—unless we persist in dooming ourselves. Quietly and effectively, over the past thirty-five years, one malignancy after another has been eliminated by our recognition of the nature of the disease and its causes.

And yet today the incidence of cancer is rising. There is nothing surprising about this, nor is it even unexpected. The increase is due to two reasons. In the first place, most of the cancers we are seeing today did not begin yesterday, but decades ago; they had their origin in the forties, fifties and early sixties. Since we know now of the lag time in cancer production, we can no longer plead ignorance. With the knowledge at hand, physicians can say without fear of contradiction that unless we take steps right now to defend ourselves, the incidence will continue to rise in the decades to come.

It seems as if we can expect no vaccines to help as in our fight, or none of the tools from the well-stocked arsenal of the infectious-disease experts. The idea that the majority of cancers are caused by viruses is currently coming under attack. Recently in the journal *Science* Dr. Howard M. Temin, recipient of the Nobel Prize in Physiology-Medicine and the American Cancer Society Professor of Viral Oncology and Cell Biology at the McArdle Laboratory for Cancer Research at the Univer-

sity of Wisconsin, stated in an article entitled "The DNA
Provirus Hypothesis," reprinted from the lecture he delivered
in Stockholm, Sweden, on December 12, 1975, when he received the prize:

"The majority of human cancers are not caused primarily by
infectious viruses like RSV, but by other types of carcinogens,
for example, the chemicals in cigarette smoke. These nonviral
carcinogens probably act to mutate a special target in cell DNA
to genes for cancer." He ends his paper: "Finally, I have
indicated that I do not believe that infectious viruses cause
most human cancers, but I do believe that viruses provide
models of the processes involved in the etiology of human
cancer." We must apparently learn to take care of ourselves.

It must be remembered, though, that we live in a highly
industrialized age, in an age of chemicals which are touted as
the answer to our needs, real or alleged, but which at the same
time can poison us.

Where the risk of carcinogenic exposure can be proved to
be absolutely necessary, it must be tolerated. But where the
danger can be avoided, as is so often the case, where the
carcinogens in our food and in our water, in the air we breathe
and the drugs we take are unnecessary and unwarranted, where
the risks outweigh the benefits, the exposure must be stopped,
the poisons eliminated.

Today more than ever before, the price of health is vigilance,
and this vigilance means that we must recognize not only the
poisons in our environment but also the efforts on the part of
industry to resist, in the name of profit, the removal of these
carcinogens and mutagens, as well as governmental tolerance
of these efforts. How often do we not see correctives applied
after the harm has been done rather than before, and even then
only under duress!

PCB—polychlorinated biphenyls—is a toxic chemical that

has been shown to cause cancer in laboratory animals. Between 1966 and 1972 General Electric dumped some 84,000 pounds of the chemical from two capacitor plants into the upper Hudson River. When the company was found guilty of violating New York State's water-quality standards, which resulted in the banning of commercial fishing and warning people not to eat fish from the Hudson, GE agreed to reduce its discharges of PCB's to conform to federal standards, and to pay the state at least $2 million in an out-of-court settlement, *provided this sum was not considered a formal penalty.*

It was not until years after Red Dye # 2 had been shown to be carcinogenic that the Food and Drug Administration banned its further use, at the same time allowing foodstuffs already produced that contained the substance to remain on the shelves and continue to be sold.

There are no longer any cancer deaths among workers from exposures to radium. It appears now to be the plutonium workers turn. A recent government survey showed that the death rate from cancers occurring in plutonium workers was almost twice as high as the cancer death rates of all white males. Only a relatively small number of American workers are currently exposed to plutonium, but with the need for more plutonium to fuel more reactors, the numbers exposed will surely go up. Some of the workers who have already died were apparently exposed to as little as 600 billionths of a gram of the metal. Dr. Sidney M. Wolfe, the health research official who undertook the study of the government's statistics, reported that the present allowable exposure level "may be more than a thousand times too high for adequately protecting workers."

Following the discovery in 1929 of the first deaths from bone cancer in the radium dial painters, Dr. Harrison S. Martland, a medical examiner of Essex County, New Jersey, and the pathologist who first described the dangers of the almost undetectably minute amounts of radium ingested by the New

Jersey watch workers, concluded at the end of his now famous
1931 report dealing with the development of those cancers
that at the very minimum it would be crucial in the future to
have proper medical supervision over the use of radium and
X-rays for therapeutic purposes and for the protection of workers to have governmental control over industries and occupa-
tions in which exposure to radioactive substances took place
and that, finally, in his own words, written almost half a century ago, "If in a certain industry the exposure cannot be
reduced to a safety minimum, the procedure in use should be
given up for some other method; [and] if this is not possible,
the industry should be discontinued." It is as if we have learned
nothing.

In April 1976 the FDA offered to sell a list of nearly two
thousand drug products containing chloroform, a chemical
found to cause cancers of the kidney and of the bladder in
laboratory animals. The agency had originally proposed an
immediate ban on these products, but decided instead not to
recall those already on the market, while delaying the ban for
at least ninety days.

The concerns continue. With more and more women working in chemical factories, the risk of toxic exposure leading to
congenital defects is added to the risk of cancer, the need for
prevention is even greater. The number of these working
women at risk during their reproductive years is now estimated
at over one million, while young girls beginning to smoke in
record numbers and still in their reproductive years run a
continuing risk of giving birth to prematures.

This is no small problem. The mothers of thalidomide babies, of sons and daughters dead from radiation-induced thyroid cancers, the mothers of Mongoloids and children born
with cleft lips and palates attest to the dangers of mutagenic
exposure during pregnancy.

It goes on. Despite the Surgeon General's warning that

cigarette smoking is dangerous to our health, more cigarettes are being sold today to women and to adolescents than ever before.

It is obvious that if we want our children to inherit a sane and healthy world, we must begin taking care of them today. The struggle for their survival is our greatest battle, a struggle no longer against nature, but rather against ourselves.

About the Author

Ronald J. Glasser, M.D., was born in Chicago, Illinois, and graduated from Johns Hopkins Medical School in 1965. He was intern and resident in pediatrics at the University of Minnesota Medical school (1965–1968) and passed his specialist board in pediatrics while serving as major in the U.S. Army Medical Corps stationed in Japan. Returning to Minneapolis in 1970, he was on the staff of the Hennepin County General Hospital and an assistant professor in the Department of Pediatrics at the University of Minnesota Hospitals. The following year he began a National Institutes of Health Research Fellowship in pediatric kidney disease. At present he is an instructor in the Department of Pediatric Nephrology at the University of Minnesota Hospitals and lives in Minneapolis.

Dr. Glasser is the author of the widely praised book *365 Days*, published in 1971, an account of a tour of duty treating soldiers in Vietnam, which won the *Washington Monthly* Political Book Award and was translated into eight languages; the world-wide best-selling novel *Ward 402*, published in 1973; and most recently, *The Body Is the Hero*. In addition, his writing has appeared in magazines and newspapers all over the country, including the *Atlantic, Harper's* and *Washington Monthly*.